**ADAM: THE STORY OF A BOY
WITH LEUKAEMIA**

In November 1983 Katherine Adair's son
Adam became unwell. At first she thought it
was a common childhood complaint such as
measles or mumps but tests revealed a far
more serious disease. Adam was diagnosed
as suffering from acute lymphatic leukaemia.

ADAM is Katherine Adair's diary of the
time from that first frightening diagnosis to
Adam's death one year later. Written as it
happened the book is untempered by
hindsight and is an honest record of
Katherine Adair's feelings throughout this
period. It details the difficult times — Adam's
initial fight for life through the acute phase of
the disease, the courses of chemotherapy
and radiotherapy, the hospital visits, the
moments of sadness and frustration — yet it
captures also moments of intense happiness
as Katherine and her son make the most of
the time they have left together.

Katherine Adair is a pseudonym.

Adam: The Story of a Child with Leukaemia

Katherine Adair

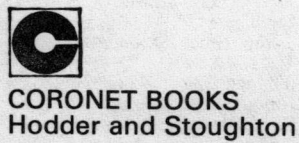

CORONET BOOKS
Hodder and Stoughton

Copyright © 1987 by Katherine Adair

First published in Great Britain in 1987 by Hodder and Stoughton Ltd

Coronet edition 1989

This book is sold subject to the condition that it shall not, by way of trade or otherwise, be lent, re-sold, hired out or otherwise circulated without the publisher's prior consent in any form of binding or cover other than that in which it is published and without a similar condition including this condition being imposed on the subsequent purchaser.

No part of this publication may be reproduced or transmitted in any form or by any means, electronically or mechanically, including photocopying, recording or any information storage or retrieval system, without either the prior permission in writing from the publisher or a licence, permitting restricted copying. In the United Kingdom such licences are issued by the Copyright Licensing Agency, 33–34 Alfred Place, London WC1E 7DP.

British Library C.I.P.

Adair, Katherine
 Adam : the story of a child with leukaemia.
 1. Leukaemic children - Personal observations
 I. Title
 362.1'989299419

ISBN 0 340 42845 7

Printed and bound in Great Britain for Hodder and Stoughton Paperbacks, a division of Hodder and Stoughton Ltd., Mill Road, Dunton Green, Sevenoaks, Kent TN13 2YA.
(Editorial Office: 47 Bedford Square, London WC1B 3DP) by Cox & Wyman Ltd., Reading.

To all the brave children I have known and those I have not known; to all the parents with an aching void; to the staff on 4B and the doctors who provide such loving care and support; and most of all to Adam, who gave me so much.

To preserve the privacy of those involved, the author has changed the names of people mentioned in the text.

1

Friday 4 November, 1983
Things are happening too fast for me and it's all unbelievable. Maybe writing it down will help me to accept what is happening and get a grip on myself so that I can help my poor Adam. Can't sleep so might just as well pass the night writing things down. Recap: Adam seemed a bit dozy and off his food for a few days, the glands under his ears were enlarged. I thought he would develop flu or some childhood complaint in a day or so but he didn't. Rang the school to see if anything was going round: nothing.

Last Sunday he raked up two trailer-loads of fallen leaves from the lawn – now that takes a lot of energy – so he could then drive the baby tractor and tow the trailer up to the orchard to dispose of them. He ate well but spent the rest of the day quietly playing with his Lego and watching television. I suddenly thought, if he isn't hatching anything obvious, maybe he has glandular fever, so on Monday I took him to the Health Centre, explained that he was off-colour with nothing very specific but had enlarged glands, please would the doctor take a blood sample to ascertain whether or not it could be glandular fever. Nicholas Peters checked him over thoroughly, agreed it may well be glandular fever, and had a blood sample taken. Enough was taken to test also for his Epilim level – I've found that he isn't always swallowing the tablets I put into his mouth for his petit mal, although he doesn't seem to be having more turns than usual. So maybe, if the dose can be reduced, he will swallow the tablets he is supposed to be taking instead of hiding them under the bed, and we'll all know where we are. Dr Peters told me to phone the Health Centre at the end of the week for the results of the tests.

On Tuesday, Adam loafed around not doing much but surrounded by Lego. We made things, periodically.

Wednesday 2 November
I had promised to take Victoria to Gerrards Cross to stay for the last few days of half-term with her boy-friend Justin at his grandparents' home. Adam is unwilling to come, extremely bad-tempered, but I can't leave him behind on his own. He doesn't tell me he isn't feeling well. He's reluctant to dress, so I help him. He strips off his pyjamas and I hand him his clothing, item by item, and sweet-talk him into putting it on. There isn't a mark on him.

On the way we look at a few shops in an unsuccessful attempt to choose Victoria a birthday sweater. Adam doesn't want to wait in the car playing tapes, he trails along with us, behaving very badly and trying to trip me up. I think he feels Vicki is getting too much attention.

After dropping Vicki off, Adam and I go on to Karen's for lunch. He suddenly turns very pale, briefly goes faint and wobbly. I'm sure it's glandular fever. He drinks three glasses of coke but won't eat any lunch. He notices a few little red spots like tiny blood blisters around his ankles; they were definitely not there this morning. I am concerned but not really worried. The doctor checked him two days ago.

About halfway through our 40 mile journey home, it dawns on me that this child is rapidly becoming *ill* as opposed to merely unwell. Instead of going home I drive straight to the Health Centre. As we don't have an appointment I ask in a loud voice, Please could someone identify this rash for me – always a good way to gain attention in a crowded waiting room.

The nurse comes smiling into the treatment room. While she is looking at the rash Adam goes white and wobbly again, and she fetches in the senior doctor. He says I was right to bring Adam in, that we should see our own doctor who isn't in the Health Centre just now – he may have heard something helpful about the blood tests, would certainly want to see us again and may want other tests done. He thinks Adam will be all right overnight, so could I bring him in to see Dr Peters in the morning. If I am worried about anything in the night, not to hesitate to ring and a doctor will come out. His manner is so calm and authoritative that it all makes sense at the time, but as soon as I am back in the car with Adam I wonder why on earth I might need a doctor in the night . . .

When we get home I settle Adam in front of the television, hug him and go out to put the bantams and ducks to bed. Almost as I step back into the house Nicholas Peters arrives. It's 4:20. He hadn't been in the Health Centre because he'd been calling here. He tells me the path. lab. isn't happy about the blood sample, and they want Adam in the John Radcliffe Hospital now. *Now?* Yes, now. They need to get cracking straight away. It's obvious that Adam has a serious blood disease, and they want to eliminate the possibility of leukaemia. *Leukaemia – Adam?* These things only happen to other people. Everything spins round. He is so kind and thoughtful – he'd sat me down in a room well away from Adam, and watched me closely while he told me all this. Leukaemia was only one of the possibilities, it *is* now curable . . . But leukaemia, my Adam . . .

When my mind stops freewheeling, I find a map and he shows me how to find the hospital. He then explains to Adam about going into hospital to have his red spots looked at. (Terrifyingly, they are now no longer only on his feet and ankles.) Adam accepts this as perfectly logical and is very matter of fact about it.

Make Adam a fluffy milkshake. I'm still shaking, grateful to have practical things to do before I start driving.

While he feeds Sheba and Cat, I phone George in the office. How do you break that sort of news gently? I try, but he cries, desperate gulps which I can't echo because I don't want to frighten Adam. Oh no, no not Adam, not my Adam he wails. As soon as you get back from the hospital please ring me straight away, I'll be in the London flat all evening waiting to hear from you, he says.

He doesn't offer to come home and it doesn't occur to me to ask him to.

Adam and I go upstairs to pack him up a few things and discover Sheba has been sick in his room. We ignore it and set off in the dark and pouring rain to find the John Radcliffe. Reflecting lights dazzling; windscreen wipers' regular beats; the sound of intense concentration; inside my head over and over again, Please God take care of Adam, Please God don't let him be hurt, Please God take care of Adam . . .

The hospital was a most bemusing complex and I discovered later that I'd parked in entirely the wrong place and was lucky not to have been towed away. We find Ward 4B just before 6:00 and I help Adam settle in a room of his own. The nursing staff are lovely – friendly and helpful to mothers as well as to children. I help Adam have a bath, as apparently he won't be allowed out of his room from now on. Someone brings him toast, orange juice and a television set.

I meet Dr Shaw, who asks what I understand to be the reason for Adam's admission to hospital. I say Probable leukaemia; he says Yes, that is what we're worried about. Where is your husband? Explain that George lives in London during the week, comes home at weekends, and yes, I have told him. The word leukaemia is never mentioned in front of the children. It *is* now curable. There are other (unspecified) possibilities. What does Adam think he is here for? I explain that he is brain-damaged, so although he is 13 his grasp of things is probably more that of a five or six year old. He is satisfied with the idea that he is here to have his red spots looked at. He's been in hospital before and isn't worried.

I tell the doctor that he's taking Epilim – or rather, should be. I'd taken his tablets in with us and ask if it'll be compatible with the medication they will give him.

Adam is settled in quite happily, bottle and bedpan to hand, television on, the bell near him. He sends me off to see to the animals – Sheba's only had a little walk today, he says. They've told me I can stay in the hospital too, but we live only 15/20 minutes away and when Adam's been in hospital before (for tests, in London) I've slept elsewhere and been with him during the day, so that seems to him to be the normal thing to happen.

Somehow I find my car and drive home. It's 9:15, and I go next door and hear myself from a long way away explain to Willow and Chris that Adam is in hospital, seriously ill, it's probably leukaemia, and as I will be spending the daytimes with him please could they put the chicks and ducks to bed for me in the afternoons. They are astonished to hear he's so ill, put a large drink in my hand and say of course they'll do anything they can to help, Willow will even let Sheba out in the middle of the day, and if there's anything else I need her for, just to ring.

I come in and phone George as he'd requested. 9:30: can't get through; all sorts of strange noises on the line. Contact

Operator and she tries a couple of times without success. British Telecom are working to rule or something equally disruptive. I think maybe he's coming home, then realise if he were, he'd be here by now. Explain to the Operator that my husband knows our son is very ill and has been taken to hospital, that he's waiting to hear from me, there must be a fault on the line, what can she do? Nothing: she can't even raise the London Exchange, although she's sympathetic and trying to help. I know George would know by now if his phone were out of order and would have gone somewhere else to phone me; he suffers withdrawal symptoms if he's away from a telephone for 30 minutes.

Today started off to be so ordinary but now I'm in a state of half shock, half panic: is he lying there alone and incapable because he's had a heart attack or something? He reacted so badly when I phoned him earlier. I become more and more convinced that this is what has happened, and pace the house wondering what to do. Can't fix in my mind where various friends live in relation to George; can't remember the names of the neighbours.

After 10:30 I try calling the local police station in London to ask them to go along and break in if his car is outside. Can't remember the number of his car, my brain won't work. Can't get through anyway – I try three times. Can't stop shaking. What does one *do* in a situation like this? It's all unreal. Feel desperate, my knees turn to jelly, a big help *that* is, I'm cross with myself but I can't help it. Nothing bad can have happened to George, we need him so much. Ring, phone, ring.

At 11:30 he rings me. He has a cold, he says, feels rotten – he felt so low on hearing my news about Adam that he went out to dinner with friends to take his mind off things. I'm totally lost for words. We may not have the best marriage in the world, but this is my husband, Adam's father. I wonder if he realises how close he came to having his flat broken into by the police. I wonder what he would have said.

He says he will phone again tomorrow to find out how things are.

I have never felt so alone and so frightened in my life. I throw up.

Can't contemplate sleep, so after a painstaking cleansing of Adam's bedroom carpet after Sheba, I spend the night tidying, hoovering and polishing. Mindless activity. I clear away some of Adam's things – there's Lego everywhere, I think it breeds – and I pick up a piece of paper which flutters down from his spelling book: D it says, Dead, death. Push it to the bottom of the bin. That isn't enough: go empty the bin. This is all too theatrical to be real. Feel as though I've been caught in a horror film.

At 3:30 a.m. I walk Sheba in the rain. She's puzzled. Come back, do some laundry, feed and release the ducks and chicks, give them fresh drinking water – what comfort in routine. Later, sort out some of Adam's favourite books to take in with me, bath, dress, phone the nursing home to tell them I can't collect Grandad and take him to his hospital appointment on Friday after all, explain, cry.

Back at the hospital, Adam's sitting up looking relaxed and cheerful. I hope I am. I feel nothing can ever be the same again.

Thursday 3 November
Adam has an anaesthetic so they can take a bone marrow sample from his hip for diagnostic purposes and also take more blood samples. When he's round from that they fix up a drip and give him four bags of platelets to stop the tendency to bleed. He's not happy about this, he's terrified of needles, although he doesn't pass out as Victoria is inclined to do. He hangs on to my hand while I cuddle him and tell him how important it is and give him lots of praise. He spends a couple of hours in the afternoon yelling at me and swearing, saying he's not brave enough for this, he's not staying here, he'd rather go home *with* his red spots. I hug him when he'll let me, try to give him confidence – if I can seem serene he'll be able to face things more calmly. Read to him. It's all difficult.

I meet Dr Morrison, the consultant paediatrician, who wants to know where my husband is, says I can't go through this by myself. He says it is acute lymphatic leukaemia (ALL), there are two sorts and they'll know which type by Saturday when he'll meet George and me to explain things. A very nice man, rather shy.

Adam settles down to watch children's television, tells me to go see to the animals. I want to stay near him but don't yet know whether he copes better when I'm there with him or not;

don't want to hover and distress him. Also, I know he is very ill, the experts have told me so, but somehow I can't accept that emotionally, even after writing it down. Anyway, he wants me to go home, so I do.

Write to Adam's headmaster, phone and write to divest myself of various obligations. Cook myself an omelette, watch it go cold, feed it to Sheba, who's very grateful. Don't sleep.

Friday 4 November
I just don't relate to the world. This morning I'm amazed to see thick fog; weather is such an ordinary thing, it has no right to be intrusive now our world is upside down. Feel a trifle weak around the knees.

Walk Sheba round the fields early and almost lose my sense of direction in the fog, which covers my hair with dewdrops. Find a hedge and follow it home.

Stop to buy some wool so I can knit Adam the sweater I'd promised to make him. Drive terribly carefully. I'm on automatic pilot and every now and then something slips, as when I sat in the car park, quite unable to make up my mind which space to pull into.

I love that child so much I feel it must protect him, there can't be something seriously wrong with him. My brain knows, Yes, sure, these things happen, why not your child? Another part of me says But he's just a bit unwell, not really ill – a little medicine, some rest, he'll be fine. Look, George knows it isn't too serious, he hasn't rushed home, it *must* be all right.

I know I need some sleep.

Adam is sunny, but I'm soon sent packing while they do a lumbar puncture and of course take more blood. The lumbar puncture takes around three hours and he also has an injection of methotrexate into his spinal cavity to kill any leukaemic cells which might be there. He has to lie flat afterwards and does not like all this one little bit.

I ask the doctors if they could possibly co-ordinate lumbar punctures and things involving needles with the bone marrow samples in future, do it all under the anaesthetic so it won't hurt or frighten him. They promise yes.

Epilim won't mix with the more important drugs they're giving him so it has been stopped. He's having anti-inflammatory drugs and also a regime of nasal spray, mouth wash, under-arm and groin wash. This, and being confined to his room, is because he now has too few white blood cells and therefore has very little natural immunity to infection, partly because of the disease and partly because of the treatment. There is a chart on the wall headed 'neutropenia routine', and we tick off washes at the appropriate times. The nurses all snatch up a wrap as they come in, and call it reverse barrier nursing. The doctors don't.

After lunch Adam goes down on his bed for a chest X-ray, then fun and games with the drip which won't go through as quickly as they want.

He's pleased I brought him in my kitchen radio and requests some of his tapes. He's very pleased I've started knitting his sweater and asks me to leave the wool and the 'needle sticks' in his room when I go home. Ask again if he'd like me to stay with him in the hospital but he says, No, Sheba, Cat, the ducks and chicks need you too. I think this handful of normality is important to him in all this extraordinary business, so I go along with it, although I want to stay with him. As though my presence could really give him strength.

He can't play much because of the drip in his left hand, but we play word games. Mummy from outer space who doesn't understand what this word means, please explain. It's fun, but nothing memorable, like the definition of opera as a sort of play in which everyone got killed but instead of bleeding they sang; or being told a sweater was something you have to put on when your Mummy starts feeling cold.

I fetch bottles and bedpans, help with the neutropaenia routine, fetch drinks, read to him and, when he wants to sleep or just watch television, I sit and knit and try not to think of the French Revolution. He likes to know I'm there during the daytime, starts to worry about the animals after dark. He sleeps a lot.

George arrives home late evening. We have something to eat, I have to spend too long in the bathroom afterwards . . .

He apologises for my couple of hours' distress on Wednesday: an error of timing and too much imagination on my part, he says. He sleeps in the spare room so he won't give me his cold. I start writing all this down.

2

Saturday 5 November
Adam looks pretty rough today and was sick three times although he has an anti-nausea drug in his drip to counter the side effects of the drugs. He eats and drinks nothing. I think he looks yellow, they tell me it's because the hospital sheets are whiter than white. I didn't notice that before. The word that slides into my mind is jaundice. Maybe the doctors are better at judging hospital laundry than I am.

He has bruising today too but no more little red spots than previously. He pushes his little tractor around a bit, listens to the radio, watches television and sleeps.

George and I see Dr Morrison, who explains that there are two sorts of acute lymphatic leukaemia; the most common one has a fifty-fifty chance of survival, the other about a ten per cent chance. Next week we should know which type Adam has. He doesn't recommend bone marrow transplantation, which is a nasty business and doesn't show much better results than the drugs, but we'll talk about it if he happens to have the low-prognosis sort.

They'll sling all the drugs in the book at him for four to six weeks, during which time it is likely that he'll haemorrhage or succumb to infection. I can't believe I'm hearing this. *Adam.* Radiation therapy if he doesn't. Lumbar punctures once a week for six weeks; blood samples twice daily. Poor Adam. The treatment isn't nearly so bad as many adults think. In this country it wouldn't be possible to get into the situation where leukaemic children throw themselves out of windows because they can't face any more treatment, as happened in Sweden some years ago. If he doesn't respond to treatment they will stop it. They won't let him feel pain – now that starts a little warm ripple in my icy mind. I can't bear to see him frightened and hurting, I'm so relieved to know that if they realise they're losing they won't continue to torture him with needles.

Dr Morrison says we must tell Vicki. George's instinct is strongly protective – this is nasty news, she has two more O-levels coming up, we should not tell her. I also want her to have as good a chance as possible at her exams, but feel strongly that she has the right not to be excluded from this devastating family occurrence. We've just been told that Adam might die in the next few weeks; our minds are denying this possibility, but she *must* be told. We spend the evening arguing.

George eventually agrees to tell her that Adam is very ill, undergoing tests in hospital, and it looks serious. If she'd like to see him before she returns to school, George will fetch her from Gerrards Cross. He phones Justin's grandparents only to discover she is no longer there. He is furious, but eventually tracks her down. She is very upset at the news.

Sunday 6 November
We both go to early communion then George goes off to the nursing home to visit his father. Matron sent him to his hospital appointment by taxi on Friday. I'm so glad he didn't have to miss it, he worries so much about his foot cancer.

Adam tells me he was sick in the night. He's had no food since Friday but he manages to get some Lucozade down. George wears a mask again, he's terrified of bringing in infection. He gives Adam a get-well card from Grandad. While Adam sleeps we have a quick pub lunch and I do eat a little. Adam watches football on television while four more bags of platelets drip in. George works in a corner of the room; I knit. How domestic, how ordinary. George goes back to London and Adam looks a lot pinker.

Monday 7 November
The schoolteacher is with Adam when I arrive. He's sitting in his chair looking quite bright and enjoys playing with the electronic arithmetic toy she's brought in, and its spelling counterpart. He soon gets tired and shaky, having to be helped back to bed. He has five more bags of platelets this morning. Another shaky shivery attack – he presses '8' as his answer on the arithmetic machine and it registers '888' so the machine tells him the answer is wrong and he's bewildered. Give him Lucozade but the doctor says his blood sugar level is 7 which is apparently okay and doesn't account for the shakes. Haemo-

globin is down so they'll give him whole blood this afternoon.

While they set up the transfusion, Adam sings 'Blood, blood, glorious blood' to the tune of the Hippopotamus Song, and later talks of its being a Ribena drip – his spirits are great! We talk, play, laugh a lot. I fetch myself coffee from the machine and the plastic cup promptly dissolves as soon as I get back to Adam's room, leaving me covered in coffee and confusion, Adam in near hysterics.

Later he becomes rather belligerent, wants to go home, he felt all right when he was at home; it's all my fault he's in hospital, it's because I don't love him any more and don't want him at home. If he can't come home he wants to die. Oh Adam. I say, Why, no one knows what it's like to die. He sits bolt upright – a tremendous effort – and says, Oh yes I do, it means under the grass and no more hurting me. But he can't tell me where he hurts or how he feels and gets cross with me for asking. We both have a stiff Lucozade and cuddle. There are times in life when Lucozade isn't nearly enough.

I'm not being enough use to him. We're so close he can pick up my moods and he has enough to cope with just now without having to bear the burden of my tensions too. I determine to be cheerful, matter of fact, loving but not over-sympathetic.

On the other hand a really sick child is silent and lethargic: if he's feeling bloody-minded he must feel better!

Tuesday 8 November
Adam in his chair, bright and playing with the speak and learn machines. He seems so much better that my stomach unknots. Pauline calls to pay her godson a brief visit, and while Adam's sleeping hauls me off for a quick pub lunch. She's been to see Grandad, bless her, and he told her all about the Great Day he's planning.

I told Grandad weeks ago that although I was delighted he had found someone with whom he could have a close personal relationship, there seemed little would be gained by rushing into marriage – indeed it could be financially detrimental to Edith – so would they please consider all the pros and cons carefully. Edith's condition is such that it could be a marriage in name only anyway. He agreed, seemed to understand, but has just told Pauline they're about to get married, and don't think they'll start a family! That comment would have floored anyone other than my unflappable friend. He's 82, Edith late 70s and wheelchair-bound – in fact between them they have enough complaints to fill a medical dictionary. Poor George was most distressed to learn his father wanted to remarry less than a year after his mother's death.

This afternoon Adam says his ears feel funny; the doctor says they look okay. We decide they must feel bubbly because he's had so many things through his IV drip he's full up to his ears; we laugh. I think if you can laugh about something it becomes acceptable and you relax, feel better: tensions add up to more pain.

George rings, from a party. He keeps in close touch by phone, says he's working late and then socialising because he's trying hard to keep his mind off 'things'. I'm trying to immerse myself, to join in 'things'.

Wednesday 9 November
A beautiful mild sunny day, leaves in full colour. Saw a kingfisher by the pond when I walked Sheba early. I'm surprised I notice all this. Unless I'm with Adam and concentrating hard all I can see is the inside of my mind which is just one big agonised scream. It somehow comes as a sharp shock when I become aware of what is around me; it's an intense, painful awareness, that all this is still here.

Adam complains of babies crying in the night: why doesn't someone cuddle them better? I know the feeling, my Adam; if only I could cuddle you better. He's had *toast* for breakfast.

The doctor changes his drip from right elbow to left wrist which upsets him considerably and he tenses up, making it more difficult. They tap his wrist to bring up a vein, like a blackbird tapping the ground to bring up worms. Poor Adam, he's such an innocent, I wish I could go through this for him. *Am* I managing to support him, help him feel secure?

Dr Shaw says Adam appears to be responding well to the chemotherapy and his kidneys are all right – apparently they've lost some children through kidney infection at this stage. His chest is clear and, when I ask about the bone marrow tests, he says some still haven't come through and, as they're taking much longer than usual, he'll chase things up. He looks me straight in the eye and doesn't blink. *I know. I know.* Icy.

Adam manages, with much help, to write a postcard to Grandad. Then I read to him, sitting on the bed and cuddling him. A doctor from the haematology department comes in and confirms another bag of blood this afternoon. I say, What's happened to your bone marrow tests, then, and he says, Oh Dr Evelyn (haematology consultant) and Dr Morrison want to see you and your husband this afternoon, hasn't anyone told you, where's your husband? He says they'll want blood samples from George, Vicki and me sometime, and disappears.

Luckily Adam wants to sleep, so I go along to the parents' sitting room to digest this by myself over coffee and a cigarette. Dr Morrison told us that (a) chemotherapy and radiotherapy had just as good a success rate with the good type of leukaemia and very probably with the low-prognosis type as transplantation (b) in the low-prognosis sort where transplantation may be considered, outside donor marrow is usually rejected, and Vicki as the only sibling would be the most likely donor. Possible transplantation can be the only reason for their wanting blood samples from us (c) transplantation is a very nasty business anyway.

Also, if it were good news, the junior doctors would be able to tell me – I just had good news about his kidneys, didn't I. If this news has to be imparted by the Heavies to George and me together, it must be bad. The 10% prognosis sort: T cell. But it *can't* be.

Adam is still asleep. I look at him, so vulnerable. I remember how, last birthday, he was so thrilled to be at last what he called a 'Teenangel'. The inside of me is screaming and icy again. Please, God, not just yet. Please don't let him be a Teenangel yet.

He wakes up hungry, wants me to fetch him a ham roll. *This* is real, a rather cross presence demanding a ham roll – the other thing can't be true, it's all in my head, I haven't been eating enough and I'm having hallucinations. But I know, really.

I read to him while the whole blood goes in. When he turns sleepy again around 4:30 I go for more coffee and when I return he's lying sobbing to a nurse because he had another injection in his leg and I wasn't there. Cuddle him. I wasn't there when he needed me, the *instant* he needed me, what sort of mother *am* I for heaven's sake. Cuddle, wash his face gently, cuddle; gradually he relaxes. Tell him that if he wants me at any time when I'm not in his room he should tell a nurse and if a nurse isn't there he should ring the bell. He knows about the bell but hasn't used it yet. Cuddle him, love him – try to infuse him with love, a sort of mental drip, and soon he stops crying. He's still very weak and would rather I held a glass for him to drink from, or fed him, than do it himself. Doesn't want the radio, or to play, even I-Spy. Just me, and then children's television.

He tells me when he thinks I should go home, as usual. He settles to sleep. I go. There are two of his favourite tapes in the car still. I play Tchaikowsky's 1st Piano Concerto, with Beethoven's 5th on the other side, over and over as I drive between hospital and home: I'm not yet ready for Star Wars.

Matron of the nursing home rings about Grandad, who's worried about Adam, won't eat or socialise, is generally working himself up. She's told him basically that the best thing he can do is to eat well and do as he's told so he'll keep fit (relatively) and I won't have to worry about him as well. All he knows is that Adam is in hospital having tests, and as that has happened on several occasions before it shouldn't worry him unduly. She's primed Edith to get him talking about other things, says he seems to have responded well today. I thank her. I've written to him a couple of times, but not been in to see him. Poor Grandad must be feeling neglected.

George phones on his way out to dinner. I don't mention my suspicions. I didn't see the consultants so they are only suspicions, not facts. Yet.

3

Thursday 10 November
Early this morning Emma arrives with a large pan of stew for me – how very thoughtful and kind. She's right, I must try to keep up my strength.

I notice more bruising on Adam's legs as I do his all-over wash.

Some get-well cards arrive from his class – handmade, beautiful ones – he has 21 cards on his wall now! Also some worksheets from school – he's delighted and works on them but gets too tired after half an hour.

Adam quietly tells me he's worried about his muscles, which don't seem very strong. I explain his body is busy fighting the infection in his blood which made the red spots, that is why he doesn't feel very strong. He accepts that, and wonders what his tummy thought about being sent down some lunch; is it pleased or is it so busy joining in the fight that it isn't much bothered? Say I think it's probably very grateful to receive supplies, armies need supplies to help them keep strong enough to fight. He likes that.

George phones. The dinner last night was most enjoyable and he looks forward to seeing us. He's suffering cold sweats though, maybe he's coming down with something. His secretary has swollen glands and an assistant is ill. I wonder if we'll see him.

Friday 11 November
Adam won't settle to doing anything. Nothing I do is right or helpful. A nurse tells him he has to have another injection in his bottom tomorrow and he gets dreadfully upset in anticipation. Cries, threatens escape. Try hard to cuddle him calm, and ask the nurse not to tell him in advance next time. Then, mid-afternoon, they steam in and give him the injection straight away – he's not too badly upset. Asks me if that's the last injection. I say he will probably have to have more, but

he'll get used to it and feel braver as he gets stronger. Explain a lot of people have to inject themselves every day, and they get used to doing it. He doesn't believe me. I'm not sure I believe me.

The drip is disconnected about 4:30 and he perks up – feels so much better when he's got two hands to use. He walks from the chair to the basin and back, is delighted with the accomplishment but disappointed he can't do it again. I curl up. He signs a good luck card and a birthday card for Victoria. I help him write a few lines to his class.

George arrives home late and only wants to talk about house-hunting in London which irritates me profoundly. Just now all I want to talk about is our son. Maybe he's trying to give me something else to think about? I'd like to believe that, but feel the only way he can cope with this situation is by pretending it isn't happening, whereas I need to talk about it, write about it, the constant expression helping me to accept that it *is* happening. He does suffer for Adam. He tells me he's been out every night this week because he doesn't want to be alone at home. I don't want to be alone either, but don't feel I have any choice: if I'm not in hospital with Adam I must be here near the phone and within easy access.

The Vicar called to bring good wishes from everyone. They are praying for Adam by name in Church. I'm incredibly touched.

Saturday 12 November
Sleep eventually and wake again before the birds, 4:45. Creep around so as not to disturb George, deal with his laundry, then wake him with a cup of tea and a shopping list before I set off for the hospital. Shopping lists – George!

Tremendous shock when I arrive to find Adam's room empty. Staff Nurse tells me that because the general ward is almost empty and free from infection they've disinfected the bathroom and taken Adam along for a bath and hairwash. He's very proud – Look at me, Mummy, I can walk back by myself! I'm so pleased and proud for him, torn up inside, too – this chap swam a mile in August.

He laughs a lot at Saturday-morning television and, when George arrives, is pleased to show him he can stand up all by himself.

Angela phones to say they can't make it today, a lorry-load of blazing hay on the motorway delayed them too much. They'll come tomorrow instead. When Adam's ready to sleep George insists I come out of the hospital and eat something. I do seem more able to cope with food when he's around sharing the responsibility, although I'm twitchy to get back after half an hour. George gets cross with me. He says Adam's in the right place, they'll take care of him, nothing is going to change whether I'm there or not.

Now Adam's off the drip he should drink ten glasses of fluid a day. I have a variety of juices and suchlike to offer him but he finds it difficult and is copiously sick.

Sunday 13 November
Don't sleep much and my foot is sore so I don't walk Sheba this morning, poor thing. Several people have kindly tried walking her for me, but she won't go. When 6½ stones of sheepdog decides she is not going to leave the house, there's not a lot one can do.

Adam in his chair, dozy, having enjoyed another bath. I read to him, we watch television. Remembrance Day Service. Adam asks which row I'm on – he takes a keen interest in my knitting – and then almost in the same breath he says quietly, I wish I'd died, you know. Ask him why, gently. Reply: It'd be so quiet and peaceful. Tell him dying is the one thing we all have to do at some time, but not yet, please – however would I manage without him? I'd just have to learn, he says. Have an uncanny feeling that he knows more than I do, that he is trying to prepare me.

George arrives, Angela and Alan shortly afterwards, and he brightens up. When Adam has eaten and is sleeping we go out to lunch. Although I'm uptight about his wishing he'd died, it's good to be with friends, to know they've come all the way from Somerset to be with us, give us their love.

Adam is very quiet again this afternoon but eats well, isn't sick. Puts himself to bed at 6:30 and asks me to turn the lights out and go home. He looks like a handsome bush-baby these days, with huge eyes. I love him so much. I wonder how my pain compares with his pain, and George's. How I could help George; we just don't seem to get through to each other.

Monday 14 November
Adam bathed and *dressed* when I arrive! He's mighty cross though. He says we never take *him* anywhere and he wants to come home because the doctors can't make him better – they aren't clever enough, although they're trying, and they're giving him the wrong medicine. I say, But you're feeling much stronger now than you were last week, so they *are* making you better; come on now, some worksheets, you. He refuses to work for me but the teacher gets him going on some English so I slope off to the parents' sitting room. They've refilled my favourite coffee machine – I've developed a close personal relationship with that machine.

I wonder what Adam is picking up from me to make him so fatalistic. Nothing is discussed in front of him unless it's good; the attitude of the staff is marvellous. It's either from inside himself or he's picking up my doubts and insecurities. I must try to be more positive in my attitude.

Meet a girl whose fifth child, a baby of six months, has an inoperable cancer and a colostomy, is undergoing chemotherapy. Meeting other parents who feel desperate takes away some of the terrible feeling of isolation. It seems dreadful to take comfort from others' distress, doesn't it; I wonder how the process works. I wonder if the hospital realises just how important the parents' sitting room is.

I ask for an appointment with Dr Evelyn. It's time they told me.

This afternoon I take Adam down for another X-ray – the furthest he's walked – he enjoys it! I humbly realise how interesting it must be to walk along hospital corridors and go down in a lift after the confinement of four walls. Then I read to him again: 'Do you like green eggs and ham? I do not like them, Sam-I-am.' Dr Seuss. Another injection in his leg and he isn't nearly as scared this time. More Dr Seuss and Richard Scarry till television time – we both love Willo the Wisp. He eats well. He decides he's going to sleep around 6:00 so I help him with the neutropaenia routine and leave.

It's very cold; the car next to mine is all iced up but mine isn't – aren't I lucky! Must find out how to turn the heater on. It's so warm and dry in the John Radcliffe and I can't catch cold or they wouldn't want me to be with Adam while he's so vulnerable.

Several phone calls from friends, which I appreciate but try to keep brief. Must be available. Heat myself a can of soup. Sheba eats it.

Tuesday 15 November

Happy birthday, dear Vicki. It's frosty, and I give the ducks fresh water on top of their ice, fresh straw on top of the old. I'll be sweeping dust under the mat yet.

Find Adam dressed but white-faced and silent, barely able to assist the teacher in dinosaur construction by dabbling a little Polyfilla on with his fingers. Drs Day and Keith appear and explain his temperature is up a little and they'll put the drip back up, give him antibiotics to help combat the infection. Adam very unstable while I wash the Polyfilla from his hands, I have to hold him up, then help him on to his bed. Doesn't want television, just me and rest. Cries, can't tell me why. Cuddles. It's all I can do. Poor Dr Day misses on his first three attempts to get the needle into the vein, isn't even certain the fourth time as the area is swollen. Adam is terrific, but it hurts Dr Day as well as me. He asks, How are you, do you want anything. Say, Maybe a bed next to Adam's and a drip of my own, perhaps a gin and tonic drip, but being facetious doesn't really help. Rest, no lunch.

Adam feels better before they put the antibiotics into the drip, eats a couple of ham rolls. I read Richard Scarry, sit holding his hand. The room is hot, my hand icy. Adam has that flushed and glassy-eyed look which I think indicates a high temperature, says he's freezing. Put the thermometer under his arm just as the nurse comes in – his temperature has indeed shot up. Cold baths, open windows: it goes down again. When he's ready to sleep around 7:30 he wants me to go so I do but it doesn't feel right. The nurses say, Yes, go home, and promise again they'll phone if he wants me.

More phone calls – I have some marvellous and very supportive friends – but keep it very brief. Letters, cards and notes from people. George phones, Willow comes in from next door. She's a darling, so helpful and kind. The door was open, as usual, and she just walked in. I must get used to closing it; if I were held up or raped just now it'd finish me completely.

Keep telling myself I must eat at least once a day, I do need to keep up my strength, such as it is, in order to help Adam.

It's so difficult, though; when I do eat I have to spend the next couple of hours in the bathroom so it doesn't seem to be doing me much good.

Wednesday 16 November

Adam's eating boiled egg and toast soldiers, looking so much better than yesterday and his temperature is normal too! I do his all-over wash and the neutropenia routine and he's exhausted again. Read. He has blood taken three times and a leg injection and is still friends with Dr Day!

No one can tell me when Dr Evelyn will see me. He apparently wants Dr Morrison to be there too and that's hard to arrange. Never mind; I know.

Adam eats lunch, sends me off for ham rolls and is cross I can't acquire immediately whatever he fancies to eat. No one ever takes *him* out to lunch. Promise that as soon as the doctors say he can come home we'll go out for a lovely celebration lunch.

Dr Morrison comes in, asks Adam if he's all right and explains he wants to take me off for a little while. He knows I've asked to see Dr Evelyn but he isn't there so he'd better tell me. I think, No, you poor thing, you don't have to, I already know and I understand how difficult this is for you too. A nurse is in the room, watching me with intense concentration, ready to spot imminent fainting or hysteria.

He says it is T-cell, the low prognosis sort. So far Adam is responding well to the induction of treatment, which is halfway through. He could still die in the next two weeks but they haven't lost one in the acute stage in the last six years. When he's in remission we can ask Vicki for a blood sample for typing to see whether she might be compatible as a possible donor. If she is, we have to consider that question. He would be strongly against the operation from a non-related donor; it's exceedingly unlikely either parent would be compatible. A bone marrow transplant is not too bad for the donor, a very dangerous and unpleasant process for the recipient, but it *may* raise the chance of survival to 40 or 50%. I can't think of anything else to ask. Dr Morrison is super but I do feel sorry for him too.

I'm knocked out, even though I knew already. Go along to

my favourite coffee machine, a cigarette in the parents' sitting room. I can't bear this.

Adam has a good appetite for supper – sausages and mash with canned tomatoes, twice over. I feel so sick I can hardly stay in the room while he eats. I can't believe he is so very ill – how could you eat sausages, mash and canned tomatoes when you're ill, for one thing? He settles to sleep, sends me off home.

Emma comes round – with her sherry decanter. I love her!

When George phones, I give him the bottom line and he says, Damn, damn, *damn*. As British as David Niven.

I wonder if I'll ever feel warm again.

A light bulb blows and I have screaming hysterics, all by myself, and frighten Sheba.

4

Thursday 17 November
Don't sleep till very late, wake feeling drugged, heavy, tummy in knots. Angela phones early and offers again to come and stay with me. Says if I want her just to phone, any time, day or night. Thea said the same, and Karen. I'm so lucky in my friends.

Adam shows me an ulcer on his tongue but says it doesn't hurt. He can't remember whether or not he's had breakfast. When I do his all-over wash he can stand in the bowl while I do his legs, but holds on to me and is very tired afterwards. Dr Day takes more blood, Adam's eyes are dreadful, he's tense and terrified. He retires to bed again, with more antibiotics in the drip. I ask Dr Day why he can't remember about breakfast – do the drugs disturb the brain? Probably it's just because hospital patients do get very disorientated, he says. He'll be very good, our Dr Day.

When Adam sleeps I go along to the parents' sitting room which is empty so I look at a magazine – the problem page. Am riveted by the fact that some mother can be desperately worried by her child's verrucas. Stella comes in, the mother of the baby with cancer; we hold on to each other and laugh, slightly hysterically. Everything's comparative. That child's verrucas did Stella and me a power of good.

Adam tells me this afternoon he thinks I look tired, not well.

I meet Dominic's mother in the doorway. Dominic is in the room next to Adam's, and he will be 4 the day before Adam is 14. He's been ill for three years, diagnosed ALL (the good sort) for two years and is back in hospital because he has an infection he is not throwing off. Mother cheerful, says the first three months are the worst and after that you get used to it. You come to out-patients regularly, go away on holiday (but she wouldn't take Dominic abroad), the child goes to school (but she never took hers into shops). She says it hardly makes any difference to their lives. He's little and the only child;

Adam likes to go swimming, to the cinema, to Youth Club and Scouts, to the Mediterranean on holiday, and these things are beyond her experience. I can't imagine how our life will be when Adam comes home. She agrees that the little booklets about leukaemia are so generalised they're no help. We'll talk again.

Adam has a cocktail of drugs injected into his drip, eats enormously and watches Top of the Pops with a nurse, so I come home.

Mrs Burrett calls round with a birthday card and some money for Adam; Mike brings a card signed by all the Youth Club members and the newsletter. How thoughtful.

George rings and sounds absolutely whacked, says he's finding it hard to concentrate, he's under considerable pressure, but doesn't feel he could take time off. That has to be his decision, and I think he'd probably find it a greater strain to sit in the hospital with nothing constructive to do. He says he'll bring his video down for Adam.

Friday 18 November

Arrive to find Adam furious that he couldn't have any breakfast and hopping mad that he was sitting there, hungry, but they hadn't yet taken him down for his anaesthetic. After a little Valium, he goes down about 10:30 in a wheelchair and a rather better frame of mind. I hold him, stroke him, talk to him, and he slips under very quickly. I have a quick coffee and am in his room waiting for him when he's brought back in less than an hour, disorientated, sleepy, but still very hungry. Sips of water, cuddles, lunch allowed at 1:00 – he sends me off to fetch him sausage rolls, too, which he wolfs down and then he dissolves into tears. When I ask why, does anything hurt, he'll only say, I dunno do I, and wail again, terrible sobs, and he's furious with me for asking stupid questions . . .

He has five bags of platelets (someone tells me they're £100 a piece – thank heavens for the National Health Service). More antibiotics, two bags of whole blood. He's very miserable all afternoon, blaming me for his being in hospital. He's all right really, it's all my fault, can't he come home now. It breaks me up.

Dr Morrison comes in to say hello and tells Adam he's doing well. Tells me they now know what infection he has and that he's being treated for it – disappears while my mouth is open to ask what. Do they train them to vanish like that, or does it come naturally! I know he'd tell me if it was something I'd understand.

The ulcer on Adam's tongue is better but his bottom looks sore. He's badly bruised and has lost a lot of weight – don't know how much. He remains tearful and cross with me. I feel useless and it seems a never-ending day.

Home by 8:00, George arrives about an hour later. He cooks us supper while I do his ironing.

Saturday 19 November
Leave George with a shopping list. Find Adam very pale, but sitting in his chair in front of the television. He's unresponsive, temperature below normal; very soon feels tired, gets back into bed after lunch. George arrives, gets a beautiful smile, but Adam's going to sleep so he takes me out to eat.

He enquires on our return about the video and cassettes, but the little nurse says it's not advisable to bring them in as they may introduce germs, wait for the Ward video to come back from repair. I don't understand the logic of this. Adam is allowed mail, visitors (briefly), and things I bring him from home. The doctors and nurses come in just to say hello, how are you, what are you doing, not only appearing when they have to give him medicine or something. I'm glad for him that it's like that. But I remember Brian's experimental rats which have to be kept free from infection: you can't go into their room without first stripping, showering and putting on a sterile gown. And I'd have thought the Ward video more likely to harbour germs than one from home. I'm confused. They seem only to play at keeping these children free from infection, and yet the system is more liveable that way; these are people, not rats.

Adam eats well this afternoon, laughs a lot, looks much pinker than before and becomes engrossed in television in the evening. However did they manage sick children before television – it's a godsend!

Sunday 20 November
George went to visit his father before joining us at the JR. He also asked Chris to put in Adam's new bedroom window as a

Christmas present for him – he'll be so pleased! (While repainting we'd discovered a badly-plastered area of wall which appears to be a bricked-up window, and replacing it would improve the room considerably.)

After Adam and I have done his all-over wash and the rest of the routine, nurse announces it's hairwash day and amid many protests from Himself she and I start dismantling the bedhead and together go through the laborious process of shampooing him as he lies in bed. He sits up afterwards but is exhausted by the effort involved in the cleansing ritual. I'm not allowed to borrow the Ward hair-drier for him this time, in case of introducing infection . . .

My son is very argumentative with me. I wonder if I find this easier because his understanding is limited, or not. Yet on a deeper level he seems to understand more than me.

Adam eats well. Food is very emotive. I know it's not as important in fact as fluid intake, but somehow a mother feels better when her child eats. He's still bruising, and losing weight and his hair.

Gleefully he tells me to go shopping before I come to see him tomorrow, so I have his birthday presents ready for Tuesday.

Monday 21 November
Sleep so heavily it's hard to drag myself from bed. It's either all or nothing these days. Buy Adam books, pyjamas, toys, drop them at home before I go to the JR. He's asleep so I go for a coffee, leaving my things so he'll know I'm around if he wakes.

There's a terrified girl in the parents' sitting room, her baby's in with possible meningitis/encephalitis – you can see the big question Brain Damage weighing down on her. Get her talking and I do hope it helps – at least she isn't shaking quite so much.

Stella tells me Baby Laurie doesn't have much chance, unless the chemotherapy reduces the tumour sufficiently for them to be able to operate.

Meet the paediatric social worker in the corridor. She gives me another leaflet and promises an introduction to Maxine, the community paediatric sister.

Adam eats fish fingers, mashed potatoes and canned tomatoes for lunch, following that up with ice cream, two ham rolls and two jumbo sausage rolls. Feel sick at the thought.

Dr Morrison comes in and tells Adam he's doing well. Apparently he had a blood infection, and they've changed his antibiotic.

John calls in with some cards and things for Adam's birthday tomorrow – Adam gives him a beautiful smile but won't really talk. I'm overwhelmed by the kindness of people we don't know well, haven't known long – we've only lived in the village for two and a half years.

We give Dominic a birthday card and later he sends Adam a piece of his birthday cake. When I see his parents by the door, they tell me no two children present or respond in the same way; no, you can't understand what's going on, it's always at least one jump ahead of you; to expect Adam's appetite to swing to extremes, with cravings for certain foods, as a side effect of the drugs; and that Maxine is marvellous.

Leave Adam feeling very excited about his birthday tomorrow. Spend 15 minutes scraping ice from my car with a credit card; when I get home I find a book on herb gardens for me from Emma – a present for me for Adam's birthday, as well as one for him! Whatever have I done to deserve such super neighbours.

George comes back. He's bought Adam a watch. We wrap presents together. I'm giving him a cassette from Sheba and Cat, fancifully spend ages dipping a reluctant Cat's wet paw into cocoa in an effort to reproduce a pawprint signature; it should be possible but for some reason I can't make it work.

Tuesday 22 November
Very cold and frosty as I set off loaded with presents; George stops off to collect the birthday cake he ordered and we meet up outside Adam's door. He's in his chair, not quite so buoyant as yesterday but very pleased in a quiet way with all his cards – 23! – and gifts. George takes photos as he unwraps and looks at things; after about an hour he's so tired he can hardly keep his head up. I help him back to bed, go along for a coffee while he sleeps; George returns to London.

Adam plays his new cassette non-stop for the rest of the day. I help him make up his Lego helicopter – he does very well with only a left hand to use – then he flakes out and sleeps again. Play, read to him, sleep.

Our Ward, 4B, is on 'take' and very busy this afternoon with many new admissions, but still the nurses and Dr Day come in to have a slice of cake, chat and wish him well. All dutifully admire his digital watch – he's been telling me the time every two minutes! They produce a card signed by all of them and two packages, a very large bar of chocolate and a sort of pinball game which can be played with one hand – it sends monkeys up palmtrees. It's super of them and I'm so grateful for their kindness.

He eats chicken and ham, mashed potatoes and canned tomatoes! Decides he's going to sleep, lights off, go home Mummy.

Spend 15 minutes defrosting the car again, drive home through freezing fog. George phones to see how the rest of the birthday went, from his meeting at the Inn on the Park.

Wednesday 23 November
Woken by the phone before 6:00 – terrified, sure it was the hospital. It's my mother, calling from Australia to tell me uncle died, and how is Adam. I've written telling her he's in hospital, but because of her bad heart condition I'm afraid to tell her more than that it is a blood disease, which I think sounds bad enough anyway. I'm paralysed, can't say much to her. I hope she'll start taking care of herself now she doesn't have to look after uncle.

Beautiful cobwebs and the ice on the duckpond is too thick for the ducks to break – they skate about in confusion, very vocal in their disapproval. I have to take an axe to the pond. It amuses Adam when I tell him.

Nasty crash on the A40, policemen getting in the way everywhere; arrive late. When the teacher arrives to do some schoolwork with Adam I lose myself in the parents' sitting room again. The baby with meningitis is responding, her mother is beginning to relax and rejoin the world. Return to Adam at the end of the lesson.

Maxine, the community paediatric sister, comes in the afternoon and spends about an hour talking to me in Sister's office. She's very helpful, easy to relate to. Adam will have to attend radiotherapy for two five-day sessions at the Churchill on discharge from here. Take great care for the first couple of weeks at home, then live life as normal. No need to sterilise the kitchen worktops or anything like that. Animals are okay. About six people attend Clinic each week, two are T-cell like Adam; she doesn't know of any terrible complications caused by the drugs. She says, Is there anything else; say, Well, a book about leukaemia written for a rather slow five-year-old would help me – and she produces one, God bless her!

When I go back into his room, Adam is pulling out his hair by the handful. And he noticed his drip running out while I was with Maxine, so with great aplomb he rang the bell and told the nurse.

He's apparently no longer neutropaenic so tomorrow we can stop the routine apart from the mouthwashes.

Part of me is scared stiff at the idea of bringing home the child I see before me, yet at the same time I'm elated at the prospect.

Debbie, who is back with her baby after exploratory surgery at the Brompton, is thrilled to discover the baby might have ten years of life. They'd thought two years, her heart tumour being pronounced inoperable. To learn they may have ten years of Kirsty – wow. I try to be enthusiastic too, and privately hope it won't be ten years of crises and frustrations, oxygen cylinders and wheelchairs.

Freezing fog, football crowds and policemen all over Headington again.

Thursday 24 November
Dr Day confirms that they're very pleased with Adam's white cell count, which *is* his, not from transfusions. Last asparaginase injection tomorrow and the last of the two antibiotics he's taking for the blood infection, after that the dreaded drip can come out. Adam is delighted but wants it out *now*.

He does some schoolwork with the teacher but is too tired to get out of bed today. Says though that he looks forward to meeting my favourite coffee machine, wants to come along towing his IV stand. I tell him I am positively *not* going to introduce one machine to another, start *that* and you don't know where it'll end – he thinks that is very funny!

His falling hair tickles him. Tell him it'll all come out for a while, he'll be like Kojak and that swimmer whose name I can't remember. No, he says, I'll be like Mr Burrett. He wants me to bring him in some woolly hats; I think he'd be much too warm in hospital with a woolly hat on, wait till he gets home to our cold little house.

He doesn't want to play anything, even word games would take too much effort. Just listens to tapes, talks, then watches television.

The Vicar calls, and thinks he looks well.

Friday 25 November
It's 20° warmer today and Adam has no drip when I arrive. He has a bath, so misses out on schoolwork, much to his delight. But then all he wants to do is sit in his chair.

I see Betty, Dominic's mother, and happen to remark that Adam always seems to blossom like a flower during the summer holidays, and I thought it was something to do with his being near the sea and/or a swimming pool, even if that did sound daft. She said it didn't, to her; even in the depths of winter when Dominic wasn't well they'd take him to the seaside and he'd seem better. What? Ions? Iodine? Imagination?

Last asparaginase injection followed by two hours of crying from Adam, who wants to come home. I do my best but this is terrible, and I'm not sure how to cope with it. Whatever should I do with this blessed child of mine? Reassure him, try to stay calm, cuddle him when he'll let me close enough. Eventually he recovers from his desperate tears and starts to colour a picture.

Dr Day bursts in and says, Hey, Good news – how would you like to go home now? We're both frozen for an instant and then galvanise into action – an unbelievable amount to pack up, tablets to collect and take home with instructions, goodbyes to say.

Adam chuckles all the way home in the car because he'll be able to use a proper lavatory again! We don't know what pleasures are, while we have them. He winds down the car window and yells hello as we come into the village. I'm just bursting with pleasure for him.

He makes a fuss of Sheba and she of him, then he tours the house checking things out before phoning George. While I'm speaking to George, Adam carries his heavy music centre back upstairs to his room – and he was only out of bed this afternoon!

I'm not sure my nerves can stand the speed with which things happen around here; this is almost as traumatic as his admission to hospital.

Happiness is, your own bathroom next to your own bedroom, your beloved furry purry friend sleeping on the end of your bed, and a million little familiar things which together add up to home.

5

Saturday 26 November
I make Adam his breakfast, then he scrambles into his clothes so he can come up to the orchard with me to let the ducks out. The bantams ignore their food and come up with us to have breakfast with the ducks, which amuses Adam considerably. The other fellow's grass . . .

It's the first anniversary of George's mother's death, so while Adam is watching television I go quickly up to the Church, clip around the grave and arrange the flowers I bought yesterday. Shoot back home – of course he's okay, I've only been out 15 minutes.

Start doing a little housework – it's amazing what state a hardly-occupied house can get into. Make Adam milkshakes and toast on demand.

For some reason I can't explain, I move his bed round so he'll sleep with his head to the north. Some vague notion of lining him up with the magnetic field, plumbing into unknown natural forces . . .

George arrives with Victoria shortly after 1:00. We all have a late lunch then they shop for me; Vicki chooses some wool and a pattern so I can make her a sweater when I've finished Adam's. The photos George took in the JR on Adam's birthday turn out well.

It's an odd sort of day. Adam seems stronger than I'd expected, subdued but so happy, laughing a lot.

George decides not to bring his father over for Sunday lunch, justifies by saying he's afraid Adam will pick up an infection from the nursing home. It turns out to be a good decision: between them, he and Vicki forgot to buy a joint when they went shopping!

Maxine's book, although written for children with leukaemia, is chilling. I hope no one ever gives it to a leukaemic child. It does clarify some things for me, however, and George promises to buy me a copy to keep.

Sunday 27 November

George wakes me early to see the heron, standing like a statue in the fish pond. He hops out and flies away but returns twice during the course of the morning and both children get a good view of him.

Adam doesn't rest all day. He's quiet but humorous and helpful – helps me cook, lays the table, etc. He insists we have wine with lunch to celebrate his home-coming: of course, Adam, of course.

George tells him not to bite his fingernails or his hair will fall out. He thinks that is terribly funny, his hair is very thin now and he knows that is because of the drugs, not his personal habits. He likes the woolly hat with a bobble which George gives him.

Emma's horse breaks through from the orchard into our garden this morning. George and I chase him back during torrential rain and repair the fence which George manages to lean on from several different angles in his best raincoat which he needs to wear to Madrid tomorrow. It turns green and brown like camouflage. He curses me, fences, horses, the countryside in general, but it doesn't occur to him that it might not have been sensible to wear the raincoat for that particular purpose. Calm him down, remove raincoat amid a stream of expletives and proceed to wash it. Even remember to retrieve it from the airing cupboard and give it to George, with the rest of his laundry, ironed and aired, when he leaves to take Vicki back to school at 2:30.

Adam plays his tapes and talks to me while I wash up. He wants Angela, Alan, and particularly his friend Batman David, to come up sometime over Christmas.

We watch the bantams pottering over the garden and laugh a lot about the way they stand up to next-door's cat; the way their heads jerk forward as they walk; the way one finds something interesting to eat, gives a delighted cry and the others all come running to share the bounty; how proud the little cockerel is. Adam is loving and giving and absolutely super.

We sit in front of the television during the evening; he watches it, I knit. His tummy rumbles considerably and I tease him about keeping a lion – probably two lions – inside his shirt. Keep it up as we go upstairs to bed – Come now,

Adam, no pets upstairs except Cat and that's only because we can't stop her. He giggles away till he almost cries. His tummy does sound like a couple of lions and, judging by what he's eaten today, I'm not at all surprised. These moments have been such a joy; pure happiness. I love that child so much. Aggro about George and his wretched raincoat simply doesn't exist.

Monday 28 November
Thoughts turn to Christmas: panic. Plans, presents, food, cards – nothing yet thought out, much less organised, and I'm determined this Christmas will be a good one. We have to build up memories. But all my time seems to be taken feeding things. Adam: 4 sausages, 2 rashers of bacon, 2 eggs, 2 slices of toast for breakfast. Medicine. Feed Cat and Sheba. Feed and release chicks and ducks. Go shopping (Adam waits in car), make him fluffy milkshake, pizza and canned tomatoes on return, cook up for deep freeze, give Adam pizza and tomatoes again, continue cooking, give Adam 4 chicken wings and two legs, put chicks to bed, make Adam a fluffy milkshake, put the ducks to bed, feed Sheba and Cat, give Adam dinner. Roughly. There were odd slices of toast and more milkshakes in between, I'm sure, medicine and mouthwashes too. Was it the White Queen in *Alice*, who had to run terribly hard in order to stay in the same place?

Before I go to bed, I have packed away pork chops in cider, lasagne and two different chicken dishes in the freezer. I'm a bloody miracle. No, no self-congratulations, just look at the state of the kitchen floor.

Don't think I've noted before, Adam had around four petit mal turns during the month prior to 2 November, when he was supposed to be taking 1,500 mg. Epilim daily, although his blood test didn't show any Epilim. Since the hospital cut it off completely a day after his admission he hasn't had one turn, and just now he's being friendly, co-operative, with-it and altogether a darling. I feel his body is concentrating on things more important than petit mal, or petit malfeasance.

Tuesday 29 November
Our first Clinic visit this morning. See Betty briefly – Dominic's having another bone marrow sample taken, still isn't respond-

ing to treatment. Meet Sam, who's just 13 and was on the Ward for eight weeks earlier in the year. He goes to school mornings and comes to Clinic once a month. Michael's mother has five children, including a three month old baby, toddler of about 18 months, a 3 to 4 year old – how the dickens does she manage? A loving husband?

Dr Keith takes the blood sample, we go for coffee and in half an hour see Dr Morrison who tells us they're happy with the blood test. We're to go to the Ward on Monday at tea time for Tuesday anaesthetic for lumbar puncture, bone marrow, antibiotic.

Adam spends the rest of the day telling me he is *not* going back on Monday, he's going to stay here at home. In the evening Peter brings his Atari television game over and plays with Adam – Dennis looks in to say hello too. Adam has a second supper and goes to bed around 8:00. Adam has decided he wants a television computer game for Christmas; says his Daddy can afford one if Peter's can. That seems to me to be a very perceptive remark. I'm tired but spend a couple of hours trying to write a letter of the right tone to my mother; it doesn't seem to come, somehow.

Wednesday 30 November
Adam sleepy, cross, tells me 30,000 times that he is *not* going into hospital on Monday, and he wants his Daddy to build a hospital in the orchard so he won't have so far to go. A clue that he recognises his need of hospital treatment? I say the ducks and Horace the horse need the orchard and they can't drive; it's better the hospital and the orchard stay as they are. He cries, eats less, sleeps after lunch. Spend a lot of time just being with him, trying somehow to comfort and amuse. He likes me to be there with him. A difficult day.

Thursday 1 December
Adam brings me coffee in bed at 7:45! But then he cries. Cuddle him in bed with me for a couple of hours, trying to remind him of previous anaesthetics, reassuring him, but he can't remember. Tell him I'll hold his hand till the doctors make him go to sleep, he'll feel floaty and have lovely dreams, and I'll be there when he wakes up again; it doesn't hurt. Once I'd persuaded him to dress and come out – we're running

out of pizzas and canned tomatoes – he's much better. He craves both these items at the moment although they don't normally feature on our menus. I'm glad Betty warned me.

This afternoon we walk Sheba together! Such energy. Willow calls, and the Vicar, then Adam's starving again. He's been eating five meals a day and pussyfooting down for snacks in the night. In fact he scared me rigid using his torch to light his way downstairs – said he didn't want to turn on the landing lights in case he woke me, but waking to wavering torch-light and hearing stealthy movement was frightening in the extreme, particularly as I don't always remember to lock up. We now leave the landing lights on all night, both keep our bedroom doors open, and have an agreement that he's to tell me if he wants anything, at any time. For my own peace of mind.

I've tried so hard to allay his fears about next week's anaesthetic, going over it time and again as Adam tells me he's worried but can't explain why. Inspiration while he's in his bath tonight: try to explain that a boy chimney sweep 100 years ago would have been very worried at the thought of taking off all his clothes and having a bath, because that was something he never did, but Adam enjoys that, it doesn't worry him because he knows all about it. This is perhaps a little difficult to relate to hospital treatment but we all fear the unknown, I guess. Don't know what else to say, just try to project love and confidence, keep him happy.

His bruises are going pink, blue, purple and yellow but he doesn't have any new ones. His face has filled out a lot now the steroids are bucking up his appetite, and the little hair remaining is fair baby hair. At the weekend when Victoria saw the hydrogen peroxide for mouth washes in the bathroom she thought I was using it to bleach his hair!

Friday 2 December

Adam is happy when he wakes me with coffee again this morning, turns cross and weepy over breakfast, says he *won't* take his tablets but after a good deal of gentle persuasion he swallows them, crushed up with a little sugar and water.

It's bright and frosty; he wants to go on a picnic. We pack up lunch, lemonade, a flask of coffee and Sheba, set off in the car to explore. He's singing-happy as we drive around. We watch some magpies hopping purposefully about, remember the magpies at our last house – the babies would tease the donkeys by riding on their backs, practising take-off and landing. There's something of the clown in magpies. We watch some blackbirds turning over leaves, for all the world as though they're tidying one little bit of countryside by putting the untidy dead leaves behind them. Adam is relaxed, laughing heartily. It's amazing how many small things there are to look at and enjoy, if only you're open to them. We stop in Stanton St John, walk up a track next to a field which has corn shooting through. Sheba enjoys it, she doesn't get enough exercise these days. Adam soon decides it's time to turn back to the car. We unkindly laugh at Sheba, who can't scramble back inside because I've parked on a slope. We help heave her in; picnic in the car, raucous rooks outside, hot panting sheepdog steaming up the windows inside.

Back home we clean our shoes, play snakes and ladders. I shove a few things into the washing machine en passant and suddenly it's supper time again. Whatever happens to the days? Adam watches television while I comb Sheba in the sitting room – slovenly me. He takes his evening tablets without a murmur; maybe I have calmed him.

George comes back about 10:45 after a day of meetings.

Saturday 3 December
George is pleased to see Adam has put on weight – he certainly has a pot belly and cheeks like a little hamster.

I return from shopping this morning to find Adam still in pyjamas, George complaining of cold and tiredness, the breakfast dishes not even tidied into the dishwasher. And George won't discuss Christmas plans. He maintains that as long as there's enough to eat while the shops are shut, nothing else matters. I get cross.

Help Adam do a Nativity Scene after lunch, then he and I walk round the orchard. George sleeps. The chicks accompany us, amuse us a lot. Our cockerel, from a low branch of an apple tree, carries on a lengthy conversation with one of Mr Herbert's cockerels over the hedge. Adam is pleased to see his horsechestnut seedling has a large sticky bud on it.

I wormed Cat, asked George to put her out; he didn't, she's copiously sick in various places and guess who gets to clean up. It seems I'm the only one who cares.

I'm losing my cool.

Sunday 4 December
George and I go to 8:00 communion; various people make kind enquiries afterwards.

Chris and John come for the piano later (George doesn't want it but doesn't want to sell it, so is lending it long term to Pam and John for their daughter to use.) They astonish me by simply picking it up and carrying it out – hope their backs won't suffer later. Adam went with George to fetch Grandad back for lunch, so missed the spectacle.

Grandad enjoys moaning about the nursing home, says how very difficult things have been. George tells him sharply things haven't been too easy around here either. I think it's a little like school: there has to be someone we-all-love-to-hate. I tell him firmly that all nurses are lovely and know exactly what they are doing, and think he gets the message. I don't want Adam to nurture any more doubts and worries than he already has, and am sure Grandad's are unjustified anyway.

The male members of the family are all comatose in front of the fire and the television after lunch. I wash up, clear away and see to the animals before making cups of tea and seeing George and his father off. With fresh laundry. By that time Adam is hungry again.

I felt absolutely no contact with George this weekend.

Monday 5 December
Adam and I up and dressed early as electrician due to put in some power points. Chris and Peter arrive to put in Adam's new window. Luckily it's mild and sunny, Adam can watch them making the hole in his bedroom wall and fixing the new frame. Very diverting; he's excited, and thinks I should already be making new curtains. He eats a pile of sandwiches mid-morning and has lunch three times. Chris can't believe it!

The monumental masons phone to say if I'll meet them at the Church they'll put up Granny's gravestone tomorrow. Tell them I'll mark it for them.

We have to walk all the way round to the main entrance of the hospital as there's work in progress on the fire escape. I'm sure they got the plans the wrong way round when building that hospital – whoever could have designed it so that the main entrance is up a hill and a quarter of a mile away on the other side from the car park, so that in effect the fire escape at the back becomes the principal means of entry?

Lovely welcome from the nurses – Ooo Adam, I didn't recognise you with your clothes on! His usual room.

While the nurse is doing the admission papers I see the most recent one. Under 'provisional diagnosis on admission' it says ALL T-cell. If that was so, no wonder they were able to tell me before the bone marrow test results that it was indeed leukaemia, but why so long before the confirmation of T-cell?

Got it: (a) husband conspicuous by his absence and (b) give her time to absorb the fact of leukaemia. They were being kind.

Dr Shaw takes me aside and says tomorrow under anaesthetic they will take a bone marrow sample, cerebro-spinal fluid sample, inject methotrexate into the CSF and take a blood sample. Adam's CSF has not so far shown leukaemic cells. He is not in remission, that isn't to be expected yet. I ask if the fact that he's done well so far improves the prognosis, which seems to me to be a reasonable question, but no, it's not possible to tell. His heart and all other bodily functions are in full working order, tomorrow's tests will tell us more.

Radiotherapy is prophylactic and a necessary part of the treatment, it's a fine art these days and no it can't go wrong. If I won't take Adam, he could remain a patient on the Ward and go daily from there to the Churchill for radiotherapy; if I'll take him he can live at home. I'll take him, I'll take him. Yes, give him whatever he wants to eat, even if it doesn't make dietary sense; let him eat while he can, he probably won't want to when they tail off the prednisone which increases appetite. He doesn't have to drink so much now. He should wear his watch on his right wrist on alternate days to prevent bruising.

The pre-med. is usually an injection. Dr Shaw knows how much Adam hates them and will give him some other form of tranquilliser so he won't worry too much about the forthcoming anaesthetic or no breakfast when he's starving. Dr Shaw is beautiful, with his big brown sympathetic eyes!

See Stella. She took Baby Laurie home last week but within 24 hours his temperature rocketed, he developed sickness and diarrhoea and had to be readmitted. He has to go to Great Ormond Street for further tests and treatment.

Back home alone I think, My beloved Adam has a probably-fatal disease – how can I even half concentrate on other things, caring for the animals, having work done around the house, or even such things as laundry, bathing myself? Are all these things interfering with a 100% concentration, a total commitment which would help Adam more, or do the little routine things add an element of normality necessary to my sanity in all this? My birth-sign, Pisces, depicts two fish pulling in opposite directions: that's me, I can usually see two equally compulsive courses of action and remain undecided. I'm useless.

Please God, take care of Adam, don't let him be hurt.

Tuesday 6 December

Peter's tidying the inside of Adam's new window, says he or Willow will see to the chicks and ducks if I'm not back. Tear off, marking Granny's grave en route.

Adam is colouring a picture, and has had an oral pre-med. At 10:30 we take him down on his bed, and he has anaesthetic through a mask – no injection at all. Back in his room inside the hour, allowed lunch around 1:00 – pizza, baked beans, mashed potatoes, sausage rolls afterwards. One day I must meet the hospital dietician.

See Stella. Baby Laurie is throwing up again, probably as a result of the drugs they give him to reduce his tumour.

Dr Shaw tells me Adam's blood count is okay, he doesn't need any more platelets, can come home if I'll take him for radiotherapy and bring him back to the JR on Monday. Complicated drug routine described, drugs prescribed and dispensed.

Adam eats an enormous supper of sausages, bacon, eggs, followed by around six pancakes, then goes to bed, saying he's too tired to stay up any longer. Wonder if I'm qualified to get a job as a hospital dietician.

Wednesday 7 December
Heavy frost and freezing fog all day but Thea comes through it to see us with a pink and cheerful azalea for me and a big bar of chocolate for Adam. We're still trying to get his mercaptopurine down – he takes almost an hour over it, and she's impressed with his perseverance. There were moments when I feared it'd end up on the floor.

I seem to lose my place in these odd, routineless days. Don't seem to have time for normal housework, let alone anything like Christmas shopping or painting. Something has to give.

This evening George phones from the Caprice and is cross because I tell him, under close questioning, that I think his mother's gravestone looks too big. Also tell him it doesn't matter whether or not I like it anyway, so long as he and his father do. As to whether it's well put up, how do you tell, I really don't know how to judge. It's still standing, but we haven't had a strong wind today. Of course he mourns his mother, but I think he's expending his emotional energy on an irrelevancy rather than on living, appreciating family members who need him. He hasn't yet arranged to see Vicki's school, which he was going to do last month, and he *will* keep telling me Christmas shopping doesn't matter as long as there's enough to eat, which makes me mad. If he really doesn't wish to participate in family life, but just be treated as an occasional guest, that could be arranged. Oh, I'm a bitch. Did I *say* any of that? If not, should I have?

Thursday 8 December
Adam slightly better about drinking his disgusting medicine. He colours a doodleart thing in the kitchen, keeping me company while I do chores, later helping me with the chicks and ducks. I almost wish he didn't enjoy them so much, they're an awful bind just now. But he's looking forward to babies in the spring, especially from the bantams.

Mend George's jeans – why do these things matter – and the catch on my sewing-machine case pings apart as I try to put it away. Sometimes I wonder how I dare drive: machines and I do not get on well.

Adam and I go over and over again the little I know about radiotherapy. He also asks a lot of questions about children in hospital over Christmas, and does Father Christmas still come.

Friday 9 December

The consultant and the other radiotherapy people are charming. As this is our initial visit, the consultant explains as best he can to such ignoramuses what is involved, side effects, etc. Nowadays almost no cases of sleepiness and nausea occur 6/8 weeks afterwards but some children lose their appetites and become nauseous during treatment he says and the rest of Adam's hair will fall out next week (it didn't). Our appointments with the machine are 9:30 daily except for Tuesdays when it's 8:30 as we have to go on over to the JR for anaesthetic.

I explain quietly that Adam is brain-damaged. He says that's irrelevant. I say, Oh no it isn't – he doesn't look slow in any way and if someone tells him to do something and he doesn't respond, they get cross because they think he's being deliberately awkward, then he gets upset. It's my fault if I haven't explained the situation – people are kind if you give them the chance to understand. And I don't want him upset. He looks rather surprised at this outburst, but concedes the point.

Adam has to lie on an examination table surrounded by surrealistic-looking machines for X-rays to be taken and measurements made of his head. The table shakes itself slowly up, down and sideways until his head is aligned somehow, and in the anteroom two television screens show his skull with marker lines across. Dotted lines are drawn on his face from left eyebrow to lobe of ear, and crosses on his head, in pencil, and we are told not to wash them off until 22 December.

The actual radiotherapy, carried out in a different room, is quite quick. More fantastic machinery and a tiny window through which the operator can see him. Adam co-operates beautifully and seems intrigued by the whole thing.

Intend to go straight into Thame to shop, but it's 11:30 and my son is starving – it's raining heavily too. Go home for an early lunch first. Peter tells us with glee that the weather forecast is snow for the whole country.

We buy Adam some moonboots when we shop because he says his feet are always frozen. He's pleased, but tired. It's almost dark by 2:30 when we get home, and time to put the chicks and ducks away once we have 'unshopped' as Adam calls the unpacking and stowing of shopping. Coffee for me, lemonade for Adam.

George phones this evening and we agree to take Adam for his celebration dinner tomorrow. I book a table. Briony phones to ask how things are – she's just back from China, and says Nicholas Peters returns from Nepal on Monday, he's had a month's break. Much-travelled doctors in our group-practice! None of your Benidorm.

Saturday 10 December
Adam and Cat wake me with coffee again. George returns just before lunch and approves Adam's new window just as much as I do.

Adam helps George cut up a dead tree which blew down over the orchard fence in last night's gales, and after lunch they both sleep. I clean out one filthy duck house, wake George with tea and send him off to inspect his mother's gravestone, finish Adam's sweater and then it's time for us to change to go out. Adam looks very smart in jacket and tie, wears his cap. We all enjoy our celebration dinner – Adam, quiet but happy, eats appreciatively and enormously. Remember to give him his medicine on our return, and tuck up one happy and very full boy with his Cat.

George tells me how tiring he's finding the strain of all this, says he doesn't know how I manage.

Adam's demeanour over the last week was much more mature; quiet, loving, sense of humour to the fore. He's been asking difficult questions indicating he's much more aware of the world around him (e.g. why is our government called 'Servative'?), yet he still professes to believe in Father Christmas.

Sunday 11 December
Cold, bright and frosty. Adam keen to try out his moonboots so he lets out and feeds the chicks and ducks – indeed he's even started cooking sausages before I appear downstairs; he and George have a good breakfast.

I am learning to gauge the temperature outside by the speed with which Cat, stiff-tailed, streaks back into the house after her early-morning ejection.

George fetches his father over. I try suggesting we have Edith over with him sometime during Christmas, partly because I'm sorry for her and partly to please Grandad. George won't hear of it: says he has quite enough on his plate and doesn't need any more strain and hassle. I don't quite understand why it should mean more strain and hassle, ask if he can't try to expand his compassion to include his father and Edith rather than trying to cut them out – it might help him to deal with his own pain if he could diffuse it. He doesn't begin to understand me, it was the wrong thing to say. I'm not sure I can understand me, there was a glimmer of something there, but I can't explain.

I do manage to persuade him to tell his father what Adam's illness is: I feel he has the right to know, and it'll help him to understand our shortcomings towards him if he knows the depth of our concern for Adam. One can over-protect both the young and the old. I intend to speak plainly to Victoria when she returns.

Monday 12 December
Adam thrilled to wake up to a light sprinkling of snow – moonboots, mitts and woolly hat on, he does the outside chores for me and looks for eggs while I cook breakfast.

We're through at the Churchill very quickly and up on 4B at the JR before 10:00. Nurses tell us they've prepared Adam's room, which gives us a chill feeling – we think he's just in to have a blood sample taken. Dr Day confirms we've got it right and we breathe again. Adam super about blood sample. Maxine appears and gives him invitations to the Clinic Christmas party on Saturday and the pantomime visit on 9 January.

Tuesday 13 December
Devil's own job persuading Adam downstairs, dressed, his medicine taken and into the car. When we're finally en route at 8:00 he's shaking, he says with cold, I think with fear. Says he's worried about the anaesthetic, complains bitterly about no breakfast. Once we arrive at the Churchill he's calmly co-operative once more, and for the rest of the day. At the JR, anaesthetic through a mask again, back up in no time. Dr Day tells me the results of the bone marrow and CSF last week were good.

We return to the village at 2:00, stop at the little shop and happen to see the Nativity procession from the school to the

Church, Mary riding a plump placid donkey led by a stolid Joseph, all the little characters in costume and followed by the rest of the pupils, staff and parents, all singing carols. Delightful.

Wednesday 14 December

After breakfast Adam and his moonboots stride off to see to the animals. He loves his moonboots!

The radiotherapist tells me Dr Shaw phoned to ask for a blood test – he wants a repeat of Monday's. We have it done in the path. lab. at the Churchill. Adam goes in by himself, quite blasé – I'm so proud of him.

We do a little Christmas shopping together, a start, anyway. Discover the water is off this afternoon – rush round to Willow and am so relieved to learn hers is off too, it isn't anything personal. Good excuse for not washing floors. Adam dozes on the sofa all afternoon. I keep him company.

He comes through to the kitchen later to supervise the preparation of a favourite supper, chicken livers with mushrooms. Watches me cut up the livers and shyly asks if he drinks the blood would it make his blood better. Tell him gently that he has people blood, not chicken blood, which I don't think would do much for him at all. That his body makes his blood all the time: he had enough blood when he was a tiny baby and still has enough blood now he is a big boy – isn't that something? People's bodies are clever. That the medicine and radiotherapy will help make sure his body produces good blood and zaps any baddy bits. He likes that and rushes round zapping a few baddies, but he says they won't go away.

We long for their arrival, love them, care for them, curse them on occasion, and when they do something incredibly touching and innocent we melt. We're forever saying hang up your coat, close the door, wash your hands now, take your boots off before you come in, wondering if they'll ever turn into responsible people, and we love them passionately. Then someone says in a dispassionate voice that when the time comes he'll be helped out gently and you're grateful. *Grateful*. However do you come to terms with it? I can't lean on George, he needs to lean on me. I like and trust Dr Morrison, I'm convinced he's 100% on the side of the children. But I still feel raw, inside and out. Skinless. And alone.

Thursday 15 December

Dark skies pregnant with thunder. When we arrive at Radiotherapy the consultant tells me the blood films still have to be looked at. The white cell count is up, which could be over-reaction *or signs of an early relapse*. He pats my hand kindly and tells me I will hear by phone later today whether I am to bring Adam in for radiotherapy tomorrow or back to the JR for another bone marrow test. If that is okay we still have a day in hand to finish this course of radiotherapy before Christmas; if it isn't, he'll go back on intensive chemotherapy in the JR, radiotherapy will be stopped and another course started later. The fact that he is far less energetic than last week is, as I thought, because of steroid reduction – I'm thankful he's still eating well. His face is puffy and he doesn't look terribly well.

Mind you, neither do I. My knees have turned to jelly again, I've a nervous stomach and I keep annoying Adam with hugs as I walk past him. Write a few Christmas cards while Adam watches television. When the hospital phones, I'm told they've all consulted and decided Adam's radiotherapy should continue, but to take another blood sample at the Churchill on Monday; we're to go as usual tomorrow. Prolonging the agony. I want someone to talk to, to share this with me. Wish I felt I could phone George; can't. He doesn't ring me.

Friday 16 December

Adam in his moonboots sees to the chicks but doesn't want to walk as far as the orchard to let out the ducks. Much less energy than last week. I'm so glad we had our celebration supper when we did.

He yawns all the way home from the Churchill and I tease him that I'll give him a bath and put him to bed again. Smiles sweetly and says no thank you, he'd rather lie on the sofa with his furry purry friend. Which he does. When I slip out to deliver a few Christmas cards in the lane he's too tired to come with me. Ted asks me the bottom line, kindly says any time I want to go round and talk, he's there. He's a dear. How lucky we are to live opposite a couple of doctors – luckier still that Ted has retired and is usually there even when Briony isn't.

Sheba has been driving me mad kicking her dish about and

always wanting to be on the other side of the door. She isn't getting enough exercise or attention these days.

George still hasn't phoned. 9:45, phone him: no reply.

Saturday 17 December
Adam thinks he has a cold. Has a slight nose bleed. After breakfast turns white and faint, has that expression of intense concentration that children and animals get when all is not well inside them. My insides go wobbly too. He hasn't a temperature but nevertheless I phone in and ask if I can bring him to the Ward for the doctors to see.

He seems better by the time we reach 4B. Dr Morrison examines him thoroughly, says he's okay, there is that high blood count they're keeping an eye on so he'll have another blood test Monday, bone marrow and lumbar puncture on Tuesday at the JR, don't forget radiotherapy and no breakfast. Admires moonboots, agrees I was right to bring him. He gives me confidence.

Home for lunch. Adam just wants my company, so all I do is sit with him, willing him to feel better. He keeps asking when will Daddy be here, but Daddy doesn't arrive till after 6:00. He collected Vicki from school and they went shopping in London. There were newsflashes about the IRA bomb outside Harrods, several people killed and injured, and my insides went to jelly again. After six weeks neither Adam nor I are as strong as we were. However, they arrived safely, Adam bucks up considerably and we all have a lovely supper together.

Sunday 18 December
I went to bed early and almost slept the clock round. Adam has a cold, cough, sore throat but no temperature. Not at all happy and it takes nearly an hour to get his morning medicine down him; many tears.

Grandad comes in, full of petty complaints. I'm just in the mood, so I give him a glass of sherry in the kitchen and tell him how lucky he is. I did my best to look after him here when Granny died; when he decided he wanted to go into a nursing home I looked at a lot, took him to see the one I thought best, arranged for him to go there for four weeks on a temporary basis so that he had in no way committed himself before he'd had a chance to make up his mind; if he feels he'd be better cared for in one previously rejected, just say and I'll do what I can; he's jolly lucky to have a son who can fork out for a private nursing home anyway. And (holding his hand) that we're extremely sympathetic concerning the aches and pains, and the irritations of communal living, but that he must remember old age is a privilege granted only to a few. He laughs, I give him another stiff sherry and a kiss.

Tell George afterwards what I've said, and hope I haven't been too hard on the old boy. George thinks I was most reasonable, considering the old man's attitude – praise indeed!

After lunch I take Sheba with me to deliver Church Christmas cards all over the village. On our return she indicates she has come into season. What ho.

When Adam is settled in bed I talk to Vicki, trying to explain about blood samples and bone marrow transplants. Adam comes down and announces his throat hurts; hot lemon and honey all round and we all go to bed. I think Victoria is all right.

Monday 19 December
Up and with-it early this morning although it's a dark grey day. Adam spends ages over his medicine, doesn't feel well. When we get to Radiotherapy we're sent for the blood sample – he's super again – then have to wait to see the Registrar, not particularly because of the blood sample but because Adam has a cold and hasn't felt well over the weekend. The radiotherapist says she likes to keep the doctors informed about what's going on – who could argue? Then the word comes – his blood count is normal, it probably shot up to deal with the incipient infection, it's all right now. His cold isn't too bad and he seems to be coping with it very well: continue radiotherapy. As to anaesthetic tomorrow: reassess the situation then. That's as good as I could expect. Come home and phone George, who sounds overwhelmingly pleased.

Have a cup of coffee, leave Adam with Vicki and set off to do some Christmas shopping. I'm out from 11:15 till 4:45, come home exhausted and with the car so full there wouldn't be room for another cracker inside it. I've Christmas tree and all.

We spend a couple of happy, messy hours wrapping gifts, then Adam is ready for an early bath, bed, with paracetamol and hot lemon and honey. Vicki fed him while I was out. She's very good at wrapping things too – I'm all thumbs. We go to bed as well, leaving the dining room a heap of bits and pieces.

6

Tuesday 20 December
Adam seems better this morning as we get ready early and leave before 8:00. There's only a mist as we leave home, Adam wearing anorak, woolly hat, mitts and moonboots; I'm in my grey suit, it's quite mild. Before we reach the Churchill it's pelting with rain; luckily as it's early I can sneak the car right next to Radiotherapy. He's all right going into the JR, too – I drop him and the bags at the main door then go round to park. He laughs at me as I join him with rain pouring off me.

The Ward is beautifully decorated for Christmas, Adam in his usual room. Such a little thing, such a comfort. He happily gives his cards and gifts to nurses and doctors. Adam doesn't want hospital lunch, and we're home by 1:45 – in brilliant sunshine, and I steam!

Boiled eggs and soldiers for lunch, then Adam wants to go out on his bike so delivers Christmas cards for me to John and Pam, and the Burretts. He and Vicki help me jam the Christmas tree into a bucket, bring it in and decorate it. Then, around 4:00, Adam retires to bed, doesn't feel well, head hurts but won't have paracetamol. I feel guilty about having let him go out on his bike but on the other hand it's the first time he's wanted to since October, and he was out for less than 15 minutes. I wish I knew how he feels. A mother's place is in the wrong. Or are women born feeling guilty?

He comes down again later to watch television and eat some supper; back to bed early. Vicki is surprised at how quickly he swings from being full of vim and vigour to feeling very rough.

Maxine gave Adam a beautiful pen for Christmas from all the doctors and nurses. Dr Shaw worried me a little, telling me most sincerely he hoped everything would go well and that we all manage to have a good Christmas without problems. As though it were against the odds.

Wednesday 21 December
Oversleep – seem to have developed the ability to turn off my alarm clock in my sleep. Adam and I dress quickly, arrive at Radiotherapy hardly late at all. They say that because it's the last session tomorrow we'll see a doctor so it'll take longer.

Back home, Adam takes an hour and a half to get his medicine down, says it makes him feel sick and gives him a headache. Promise we'll talk about that with the doctor tomorrow. Read him a couple of stories which calms him down, then while he and Vicki decorate the house for Christmas I do yet more shopping. Wouldn't it be marvellous, never to have to go shopping again!

Wrap Adam comfortably on the sofa in his duvet, wrap some Christmas gifts, make supper and pancakes, which the children wrap themselves around with satisfactory enthusiasm.

Thursday 22 December
Last visit to Radiotherapy and we hang around to see the consultant, who only says, Well, that's that, the JR will give me follow-up information so I won't need to see Adam again. Tell him for the last couple of days Adam has complained his medicine made him feel sick: is it the medicine or a side-effect of radiotherapy? Can he advise me or should I see one of the paediatricians? He just gives me a prescription for travel-sick tablets, we tell Adam he won't feel sick with these, but he's not convinced and when we get home it takes an hour and a half to persuade his medicine down him. He shudders so much I'm sure he'll be sick, but he isn't. I'm shaking after this, so go over and see if Briony or Ted can give me any hints on how to make the medication more acceptable to him, as it's ridiculous to get into this sort of situation, wearing for both of us and very bad psychologically for Adam. Briony is at the Health Centre but Ted is an absolute dear. He finds another anti-nausea drug – in liquid form – in his pharmacopoeia, gives me a prescription and a sherry. He makes me talk, hugs me and tries to make me cry. Tells me he has a lovely shoulder for crying on – he has, too – asks if I have anyone I can talk freely to, says I mustn't bottle it all up. Tell him that there are safety valves – as when I had screaming hysterics when a light bulb went. He says Good, but it's no fun on your own, come scream at me, call any time, Briony or I will be here and

we forget these things straight away afterwards. He's so kind he brings tears to my eyes, but I don't break down. I can't.

After lunch Adam comes into Thame with me to pick up a couple of things and we take the holly posy to Granny's grave. It rains heavily once more and Adam, dry in the car, laughs at me, dripping over everything yet again.

During my absences today Victoria, without being asked, has cleaned both bathrooms, tidied, hoovered and polished the whole house, tidied the kitchen and washed the hall and kitchen floors, God bless her. The psychological lift is tremendous.

Help Adam bath, wash what is left of his hair for the first time in two weeks, settle him in bed early.

George phones. He moves out of the London flat in January, so perhaps understandably is rather short. Angela phones – they can come up on Boxing Day, I'm so glad.

Saturday 24 December

The last two days seem to have telescoped into one mad rush. Mandy has this theory that since metrication there have been only 50 minutes to an hour, 20 hours to a day. I'll go along with that. I'm pretty sure I've gift-wrapped the Sellotape; can't find Cat, haven't made a cake or rum truffles; the turkey is still unstuffed; I managed to mislay the frozen peas; the avocados are still sitting like rocks in the airing cupboard alongside some immature Brie. All the glaze slid off the ham, which looks barely half the size it was to begin with. I haven't even finished the first part of Victoria's sweater and overtop set, so I'll have to give her an IOU for that. And oh yes, I *knew* I'd bought lavatory paper. After two days Vicki came across it – in the deep freeze.

Little Black Bantam obligingly lays us four Christmas eggs.

It's 1:45 and Adam is wide awake, Father Christmas here is very sleepy! We've tried to explain about Father Christmas to Adam: Vicki says it's ridiculous for a 14-year-old still to believe in That Myth – he'll be laughed at. Adam insists that Father Christmas is real. We couldn't shift him from this conviction. Does Father Christmas have a torch or do we leave the lights on? He leaves mince pies and a glass of Scotch on the hearth; I remember to consume them on Father Christmas' behalf . . .

It's ages before I can sneak Adam's pillow slip into his room without fear of detection – at least it *was* a pillow-slip: he told Willow he thought he'd put out a duvet cover this year! Then Vicki was only pretending to be asleep when I took her pillow-slip in: I said Ho Ho Ho very quietly and she gave the game away by laughing!

Christmas Day
Writing this by the superior light of my new bedside lamp/alarm/teamaker. It's been a very long day. Awake half the night, up again at 7:30 to stuff the turkey, Adam down shortly after. We take tea to Vicki and George in their rooms at 8:00, then have a grand present-opening session in the dining room around the tree. George and the children love the computer thing he bought them – I've been too busy to investigate its possibilities but it plays games with them. None of us manages to get to Church but George takes his father to visit Granny's grave.

Adam quiet, pale, very happy with all his gifts (including a fork-lift truck from Horace, the horse in the orchard).

We've had avocados (they did soften) with prawns and just started on turkey, etc. etc. ad nauseam when Tracy and Peter from next door come in, have a drink and play computer games. Willow and Chris soon follow and we all exchange gifts. Coming, going, playing – no one wants Christmas pudding or mince pies. Of course.

I clear up the house, which looks like a battlefield, wash up, tidy kitchen, see to the animals and walk Sheba, then I rest while George makes supper for himself, Adam and Grandad – how can they face more food? Grandad must have eaten three times the amount I did, and I'm uncomfortably full.

Am worried about Victoria, who has apparently dropped out of school and who seems to think that she can walk into a job any time she likes with no further training. Must find her something constructive to do for the next nine months, a course for at least a year from September, which won't be easy.

Tuesday 27 December
Yesterday was a chaotic scramble. Up early to see to the chicks, ducks, dog-walking, feed Sheba and Cat, cook breakfast for George and Adam. Then George kept calling me to look

at things during the morning, while I was trying to clear further debris from the previous day, prepare lunch for ten as well as amuse Adam. Vicki still in bed. Much to my relief George takes Adam to the Carol Service in Church. Vicki appears feeling faint and retires again. Angela phones to say they'll be late – thank heavens, so will I! George and Adam return with Grandad.

George says, Good heavens you aren't putting *celery* into the turkey, apple, celery and walnut salad, are you; and, Good Lord, how many is that supposed to feed, there won't be nearly enough; and where did you buy that ham, don't go there again; and, I'm not carving after they arrive; and, where are we all going to sit; and, Aren't you ready yet, they'll be here any moment. He sends Adam to fetch me out of the bathroom to watch him carve, and generally makes himself useful . . .

Try hard to keep my cool instead of following the lead of one of my predecessors here, and retiring into the apple store to attempt suicide. I wish I could relate to those I am related to.

Angela, Alan and family are all super as usual, it's lovely to see them, but Grandad is miserable. It's so hard to strike the right note of sympathy with him; if you're too sympathetic he joins in with great enthusiasm and becomes terribly self-pitying.

When the visitors have gone Peter comes in for more computer games with Vicki and Adam; George takes Grandad back to the nursing home and I clear up – it's incredible how many glasses, cups, etc. ten people can use in so few hours. Get supper then Adam and I both retire early, me with a hot toddy, determined to get a good night's sleep. And I did.

Today, 27th, is a beautiful blank in the diary. I don't get up till 8:30 – luxury. Total silence. Do animal chores, have a leisurely look at the papers, and a large mug of coffee or three, before people start stirring, demanding breakfast.

Pauline phones and asks us all over for a late lunch – how lovely not to have to prepare a meal, or even drive there and back. Enjoy seeing them, have a super lunch and come home at dusk, for the chicks and ducks. A couple of boys come in to play television games with Vicki – Adam prefers to sit quietly next to me, we do crossword puzzles and watch a little television.

Wednesday 28 December
Into the JR – usual lovely greeting from the nurses and his usual room – these girls are fantastic. Dr Morrison appears just as a comatose Adam comes back from Level 1; he says last week's bone marrow was normal but he doesn't understand the peripheral blood count being so high. I'd understood the last blood count to be normal. However. He says, Wait and see what today's blood count shows. Drs Day and Keith look in but don't tell me anything, except that Adam's to come to Clinic on Tuesday at 10:00.

Maxine and Dr Keith arrange for the septrin to be prescribed by Nick Peters in elixir form rather than as tablets which is the only way the hospital can dispense it; that might make it easier to give him his medicine at home.

Home about 3:00. Adam hasn't eaten today but says he isn't hungry. When Vicki comes in later I walk Sheba while she makes some supper for Adam and herself, then she goes out again.

Thursday 29 December
Mr Burrett gives me back £5 from this week's money for helping in the garden, saying we're all so kind he would like us to buy ourselves something with it. Am terribly touched – not many people, I'm sure, are tipped by their gardeners!

Go get books about computers, books about careers in general and working with children in particular from the library for Vicki, take Adam to spend his Christmas money which is burning a hole in his pocket: Lego, of course. Also go to the dentist to have my cavity filled – there's so much metal in my mouth I daren't go too close to any magnets. Luckily Adam doesn't need any dental work done.

Sheba seems to have adopted an alternative lifestyle – she had breakfast through the bottom of a dustbin sack, drank from the pond and came in looking like a gypsy dog.

Made more phone calls re courses for Vicki, but no replies. I guess everyone's still on holiday.

Adam doesn't seem so good today. Eats only a bacon sandwich and a yoghurt, complains of feeling cold when I, a cold fish at the best of times, feel warm. He's twitchy, too. Three or four petit mal turns.

Friday 30 December
Adam doesn't want to get dressed today. He's pale, listless, no appetite and says he should see a doctor about his cold, which certainly seems no worse to me. Offer him paracetamol for his headache, which he refuses, so I reckon it can't be such a bad one.

When I come back from a swift trip to the shops he's dressed, comes with me to walk Sheba through the fields – it's a lovely crisp sunny day. He enjoys it but gets tired far too soon.

Nicholas Peters looks in just after I've done the chicks and ducks, asks all about Adam's intensive chemotherapy and radiotherapy, asks him how he feels, what he had for Christmas, when he's next going to hospital and for what. Tells me to get in touch at any time, either to ask him to translate what the hospital doctors have said, or just to talk. He's so sweet. He said to ring and keep him informed, as although he gets reports from the hospital they are inevitably out of date by the time he receives them, and he would like to know. Adam looks very white to me, but Nick says he seems better than he'd expected.

George returns, 10:00 p.m., very aggressive.

Saturday 31 December
Little cock bantam very aggressive too – he attacks my boot in fury when I let out the chicks. It's amusing now, but it won't be if he keeps it up in the summer when I wear skirts and sandals.

George asks once again if he can bring his pot plants here, and once again I tell him he knows what he has, their size, the space we have here, the conditions the plants require – this is a dark cottage. Some of his plants are huge, but if he can envisage their fitting in, of course it's all right. As last night, he tries to make a fight about it, says I refuse to give houseroom to his plants or his fishtank so he'll have to go back to London to make other arrangements for them, okay? I don't rise to his interpretation or his tone, just say, Do as you think fit, dear. Some of his monsterosa must be ten years old and three feet across; there's a limit to the number of those you can absorb into a small cottage and I'm damned if I'm going to beg for the privilege of housing them, but equally I haven't said no. He'll just have to use his common sense, and possibly his large office. And if he has a reason to return to London he can do so without having to pick a fight as an excuse.

He's on the point of steaming out when a neighbour arrives to say how shocked he was to hear of Adam's further difficulties and Happy New Year. Give him a drink: he's a useful distraction. Odd how people who have heard through a third party tell you they're shocked in an aggressive manner, as though by not making a point of telling them yourself you've deliberately let the side down.

After lunch George and the children go into London in my estate car to collect the wretched plants and I have a glorious couple of hours to myself. Sheba and I go for a long walk round the fields, it's exhilaratingly windy and as she runs her ears billow out like sails.

George still very moody when they return, saying Adam was extremely helpful and sensible, Victoria useless. He goes on and on about how he has so many problems he just can't take any more, he isn't as strong as I am. Tell him, No, I'm certainly not stronger than he is, but perhaps we have different strengths and weaknesses, complement each other; that although Vicki isn't as he was at her age, or me, why-ever should she be, after all; and that when we find her at her most difficult she is most in need of our understanding and loving support rather than criticism; that he and I must stay firm with her, with both of them – supportive and constructive.

I'm honestly finding him more difficult than either of the children, with his why does this have to happen to me, why does that have to happen, I can't take any more. He has a headache, a stomach ache, he feels sick. Oh heavens, he wants so much sympathy. I wish I could help him. I wish I could understand him. Vicki isn't nearly as bad as he makes out, but even if she were she's ours and we love her very much and want to do our best for her.

I needed an emotional battery-recharger for Christmas.

If you can turn some things around enough in your mind you can arrive at an acceptable way of looking at them. A poor prognosis is a gift of extra time, not just a possible death sentence. Adam didn't die unexpectedly in an accident as many children who die do; we have the opportunity to concentrate on making the most of whatever time we have left together.

Tell George that we want much more of his time this year. I want us to do a few interesting trips with Adam, maybe only weekend trips, but to cram in different experiences, memories, do stimulating things with him. Days out, all together, maybe a weekend in a caravan, a boat, he'd love that. George just grunts caravans, boats on the river and picnics aren't really his scene.

Karen and Brian see in the New Year with us all and George cheers up, is chatty, amusing, good company; suffers me to kiss his cheek and wish him a happy 1984, then we rush to kiss all the children who are playing television computer games in the dining room.

I clear up, wash up, on my own as usual, before going to bed.

Sunday 1 January 1984
Start the New Year by going to Communion on my own; pray for strength to help them all. Feel very much alone.

The family cheerful this morning in spite of very late night. George goes off with Adam to fetch another carload of plants. I cook celebration duck – two ducks – with orange sauce for lunch, then hear Grandad wasn't expecting to come over today and has decided to stay at the nursing home with Edith. Overwhelming feeling of guilt once more. I should have insisted on Edith's coming over with him some time – if only I could lift her by myself I would have. I shouldn't have spoken to him so firmly that time. I've been so concerned over my immediate family I've neglected the poor old boy once more – he may be feeling very hurt and upset. Must go over and stroke his ego soon.

On the other hand it could be simply that he's coming to terms with life among the old folk, and would really rather celebrate the New Year with them. I'm Pisces, after all.

George doesn't want a sorbet after his roast duck: too much, but he polishes off the best part of a 2lb. box of chocolates. I rest while they watch television, then go to see Grandad. Victoria goes out 'to see where the local talent is'.

Monday 2 January
A wild and windy day. Collect a duck egg and a bantam egg this morning. Adam doesn't seem at all well: white, lethargic, doesn't dress all day, just lies on the floor and watches television. Doesn't eat anything till supper time, when he wants buttered spaghetti (I slide an egg in too) with tomato and cucumber salad.

George puts up a shelf for me in the porch this morning. Keeps shouting for me to fetch him things – the kitchen stool, a tape, a pencil – and I have to stop whatever I'm doing and get them while he stands there, waiting. Bite my tongue, then give him lots of thanks and praise . . .

He goes back to London immediately after an early lunch; I sit with Adam. My presence seems to be comforting to him, even though he doesn't want to play anything. Watches Spartacus, Thunderball, bath then early bed. Me, too, but Vicki is still out although it's after 10:30, curfew time, so I can't settle.

Why do I now feel more alone and lonely when George is in the house than I do when he's in London? Certain expectations I have which he can't fulfil, perhaps because I can't express them?

Tuesday 3 January
Bath early, call Adam just after 8:00 as I go see to ducks and chicks. Sheba comes with me then disappears, alarming as she is still in season. Rush around calling uselessly, can't see her anywhere. Get Vicki up, she sets off with boots on and a coat over her nightie. Adam berates me for losing Sheba, won't take breakfast or medication. It's blowing a gale, dark and sleeting, and he won't put on a sweater. I feel like screaming too. Dear Mr Burrett emerges from the rose bed and wobbles off on his bicycle to help Vicki look for Sheba – I don't know where he's going or why, but have long accepted that information passes by osmosis in this part of the world. They return, Vicki with a very dirty and dishevelled Sheba, and I don't like the smirk on her face. Sheba's, I mean.

Adam thereupon takes his medicine and we go to the JR. Fire escape entrance open, thank goodness. Blood samples taken from Adam and me. Dr Keith and a doctor from haematology tell me Adam's lethargy could be a reaction to radiotherapy, all take it differently, and although they said 6/8 weeks for the sleepiness it could well be now, just two weeks later. He'll probably get stronger within the next month or so, be able to start school after half-term.

I explain about the petit mal turns and ask if maybe one of the drugs they use in intensive chemotherapy has an anti-convulsant property; they say, very interesting, maybe. He is now in remission; if he has a relapse it's unlikely they'll be able to pull him out of it, being T-cell and a boy. Blood tests weekly and frequent bone marrow tests will tell them whether he is bearing up under medication or relapsing. A lung infection which sounds like a chicken disease, pneumono-something, is to be dreaded. Blood sample from Vicki next Monday.

Adam has vincristine injection. I'm getting the hang of maintenance treatment now; each month there's a vincristine injection into a vein (which must be given by a doctor) and a five day course of prednisone which is a steroid. Once a week there's a dose of methotrexate. Mercaptopurine and septrin (a wide spectrum antibiotic) are daily, along with Stemetil, the optional anti-nausea syrup. Each drug hits the leukaemic cells at a different stage of development. I'm too busy absorbing information, I'm ashamed to say, to ask what his blood count is. They do tell me however that when they say 'normal' they mean what they would expect bearing in mind the medication, not you-and-me-normal. They take the white cell count down as far as they dare with drugs which increases the risk of infection, hence the antibiotic.

Medication at home is still difficult, even with the septrin in syrup form. Tonight I have to give him 24 tablets as well as the septrin and Stemetil. Collect some raspberry ice-cream syrup and crush the tablets into a little of that but he still takes ages to swallow it, shudders and retches.

The wind howls, the sleet sleets horizontally and Vicki still feels it necessary to go to Youth Club with Peter. I'm so glad I'm not 17.

7

Wednesday 4 January
It takes a lot to get this family up and moving this morning. I've done the chores and called the children several times before there's a whimper from upstairs, and it's 11:00 before Adam's taken his medicine and a bacon sandwich in front of the fire. He used to like his bacon crispy, now decides he doesn't like 'stiff' bacon.

Talk to Victoria, who's very positive about what she does not want to do, absolutely without ideas as to what she does want to do with her life. Get a trifle sharp.

I wonder, is George so miserable and helpless just because he thinks I am coping well, and if so should I stage a collapse for him to put together again? If I did, could he? He is a constructive and positive person but he simply isn't producing. I find it difficult enough to come to terms with me, let alone four others with sensitive egos.

Thursday 5 January
The words keep going through my mind, 'Because it's T-cell and he's a boy' the chances of pulling him through a relapse aren't good. I suppose it's because the leukaemic cells invade the testicles, can't think of anything else.

Victoria goes off to the library by herself to investigate careers and courses – am elated she's taken the initiative.

Adam's torture by medicine continues. He doesn't dress again today, we slug it together in front of the fire talking, playing quietly. I've little stamina too.

Thought: this is rather like being in labour, you have to look at it positively and work hard; if you just lie there it hurts more. Maybe that's why George is suffering so; he can't join in constructively. But I don't know why not. Don't think I can stage a collapse yet, there's too much to do.

Friday 6 January

Twelfth Night. Vicki gets Adam interested in sticking stamps into an album, undresses the tree while I shop. Then she goes in to the Thame Careers Guidance place, comes home with a YTS application for Mothercare and Selfridges in Oxford, a bus timetable etc. Am most heartened. Even Adam feels brighter, has a mug of consommé for supper (no lunch).

Saturday 7 January

A great day! Adam dresses, comes with me to feed the chicks and ducks, then has two bacon sandwiches and takes his medicine straight away! He obviously feels a lot better. If not exactly overwhelmed, I am definitely whelmed. Vicki encourages him to write in his Snoopy diary each day; he does that and starts insulting me again – he is feeling better! He even goes off on his bike, but returns almost immediately because it's too cold, creeps into the bottom of the airing cupboard the better to warm up. He feels the cold much more now.

Victoria goes out to borrow a Mothercare catalogue so she can do a little homework before her interview, and comes back with three boys in tow. Irreverent thought: should I spray my daughter with Sheba's anti-mate before she goes out!

George returns with the rest of his plants; he has taken a flat for three months and moves in on Wednesday. He's not as uptight as before but fairly non-communicative.

Sunday 8 January

If I'd realised George was leaving at 10:30 a.m. I'd have made a real effort to stay up and talk last night. On the other hand, while I was around he was busy reading things, communicating with occasional grunts, so I *won't* feel guilty for going to bed early.

This morning he tells me people in Australia are doing bone marrow transplants from outside donors with great success, and he's getting further information with a view to sending Adam and me there for an operation. My gut reaction is very strongly negative. I do not believe the Australians can do anything our own doctors can't, and I do not want Adam and me transported to the other side of the world for such treatment – we should be here, in our own environment, guided by people we know and trust, within reach of friends, easily available for follow-up checks afterwards.

I wonder whether it's possible to culture bone marrow? Could they take some from Adam, kill all the blasts, breed the good cells and put it back in such a massive quantity that his own immune system would kill any cancer cells which may remain? I'm good at having theories on subjects about which I know absolutely nothing: that way you aren't inhibited by preconceptions.

Poor Adam wonders whether he needs glasses because his 'brain and eyes' hurt, his arms and legs too. But he won't have any paracetamol, or even hot-water bottles to ease the aches and pains. He seems fairly with-it. Vicki comes in with Martin, Peter comes in too and they make snap-together trucks.

Monday 9 January

Day starts well with news of a job interview for Vicki at Selfridges on Thursday.

Victoria and Adam both have blood samples taken on 4B. Dr Shaw says Vicki didn't like it one little bit and they had to revive her with orange juice, but she didn't quite faint. She's terribly uptight afterwards, poor dear. We have lunch on Level 3; Adam just has a yoghurt and feels sleepy. The wait from 12:30 to 2:00 when the coach leaves for the pantomime visit seems interminable to us all.

It's Norman Wisdom in Robinson Crusoe. Adam complains it's too loud, rests his head on my shoulder but joins in and laughs a lot. He needs cuddling in the coach back to the hospital, sleeps in the car on the way home, arrives starving – fish fingers, chips and onion rings twice over and there are times when even instant food just isn't fast enough.

Tuesday 10 January

We expect a short Clinic visit today because his blood sample was taken yesterday. However Maxine says he's anaemic, will we come up to the Ward and arrange for a transfusion, two units, it'll take about six hours. Dr Shaw takes another blood sample for cross-matching and tells us we can get lost for a couple of hours if we want, so we come home with the intention of leaving Adam to have lunch with Vicki. However he doesn't want lunch, comes with me instead; bank, supermarket, frozen food centre, home to unload and leave Vicki to unshop while we go back to the JR.

They have the blood ready and Adam is very good while the IV is set up in the treatment room, then he's trundled out into the Ward opposite Dominic, whose transfusion started at 12:00. They brought a picnic and Dominic is bright as a button. Adam just lies on his bed, doesn't even want me to read to him.

Carol the play lady comes to offer him things and talk. She says if Vicki wants to spend time with her, finding out about being a nursery nurse, she'd be happy to see her at any time – she's worked as a private nanny as well as a nursery nurse and play lady.

The first unit of blood goes in with no problems; halfway through the second unit the blood goes bubbly so we call a nurse who squeezes the bag a few times. That seems to work, then when it stops again and she repeats the process the bag bursts and there's blood everywhere. She's covered, the bed, the floor – Adam enjoys that very much! She puts up saline and sends for more blood but before it arrives Adam develops large angry red areas on his forehead, chest and back. She starts taking temperature, pulse and blood pressure every few minutes and sends for the duty doctor, who says Adam must stay in overnight and she'll be along soon. Find Adam some Ward pyjamas, move him to 'his' room, complete admission papers, discuss his medication – they have everything here except his septrin and Stemetil which are at home but the nurse can't even give him the stuff that is here until a doctor signs for it. Dilemma.

However, when the doctor finally arrives at 9:00 she says he can go home. Drip removed, Adam delighted, dressed and ready to leave quick quick – he *likes* lady doctor!

Vicki a little uptight when we get home at 9:30, says she doesn't like to be alone in the house after dark. Explain what happened, explain that, although very old, this house is certainly not haunted – it would be rather fun I think to have a ghost but all we have is central heating with personality. Smooth ruffled feathers, feed and medicate my son, fall into bed.

8

Wednesday 11 January
Turn the alarm off in my sleep again and don't regain consciousness till 9:30. Have 10:30 appointment with Adam's new head teacher. Wake children, give Adam his medicine and a bacon sandwich, ask them to see to the chicks and ducks for me and shoot off to Aylesbury.

Head teacher charming, helpful and considerate. She thinks, as I do, that in the circumstances Adam's education would best be furthered by experiences, rather than rushing to a return to formal schooling which might present unacceptable hazards, although the psychological benefit cannot be ignored. She feels they could not offer an acceptable standard of supervision for so vulnerable a child, but they would do anything to help. And they could arrange for him to have home tutoring when I think that appropriate.

Rescue a lady who has run out of petrol, drop off a note to Nick Peters requesting a further septrin prescription en route home, and return to find no one has let out the chicks and ducks. I'm cross.

Drop Vicki off for her bus to Oxford, then spend the afternoon cuddling Adam, going through old photographs with him in an effort to convince him he was *just* as beautiful a baby as Baby Laurie. He isn't convinced and wants to change his name to Laurie.

Vicki's interview at Mothercare seemed to go well and she's all set for tomorrow at Selfridges. Adam lends her his new alarm clock as I'm proving unreliable about waking. I'll have to revert to my old trick of drinking two glasses of water last thing at night, thus engaging the co-operation of my bladder in waking me.

Adam sees Willow's two cats in our garden and remarks that he wishes we had a spare cat, like Willow. I like it!

Thursday 12 January
Didn't sleep till after 4:00, up at 7:00 to drive Vicki to her bus. Adam gets up and comes with us. Sunny, black ice, a car in the hedge by the two bridges.

Adam decides it's a picnic-in-the-car day, so we go off to buy picnic food – and duck food, cat food, dog food . . . And we stop at the Health Centre to collect the prescription; they ask me to wait, Dr Peters wants to see me.

He asks how Adam is, and tells me re the prescription request that I must not apologise for asking anything of him, it isn't bothering him, I can ask anything, at any time. He sounds quite cross. And I'm to come in and talk to him whenever I want to. He's great and it gives me a shot in the arm just to know he's there. I tell him I'd like to come and talk to him when we get the compatibility test results and discuss transplants, so he wants to talk about that for a bit. Tell him about George's Australian idea, how I can't believe they can do things out there that our own doctors here can't do, how I feel strongly against taking Adam 'doctor shopping' to the other side of the world. He agrees. Tell him my bone marrow culture theory, that I'm disappointed I haven't made a medical breakthrough and make him laugh – he thought it was a good idea too! He gives me just a week's prescription. I think he wants to keep an eye on both of us. It makes me feel warm.

Adam, Sheba and I set off for our picnic. First of all I miss the turning to Rycote, then I can't find Brill windmill. How can anyone miss a windmill – they're big enough, and must be high on the windy side of the village. Takes talent. Makes Adam laugh at me.

We watch a pair of magpies, watch some sheep, see a kestrel hovering, hovering – pounce! and speculate about its prey. Adam plays his tapes in the car, we eat our picnic. Eggs are a problem: he insists on hardboiled eggs with every picnic. Mandy's eggs are so fresh – you usually have to move the hen to reach them – that they don't peel satisfactorily; supermarket eggs peel nicely because they're stale but don't taste so good for the same reason and he won't eat them. Catch 22. We admire the shape of the naked trees, the patterns they make against the sky. We take Sheba for a walk, a short one; all too soon Adam is tired, cold. We've enjoyed our little outing though.

Adam is very sleepy when we get home. Cuddle and read

to him. Vicki goes next door, reappears to ask if we knew Willow has puppies – Adam instantly revitalises and disappears for the next two hours! So I do some sketchy housework.

Mothercare lady phones Vicki to offer her the job, says they usually need two interviews but they were very impressed with her, and they'll teach her to unfold pushchairs and measure pregnant ladies for maternity bras. She says, Thank you very much indeed, but may I discuss it with my parents and let you know on Monday. Selfridges and the Careers lady should ring tomorrow so it'll all sort out. I'm so pleased with her. Martin and Peter will help her restore the old bike.

Friday 13 January
Adam stays in bed dozing and listening to the tapes Peter lent him so I take him his bacon sandwich up at 9:00 then it takes me till 11:30 to give him his septrin. He doesn't want any lunch. He starts coughing.

The lady from Selfridges offers Vicki the job without another interview too. She phones Mothercare to say, Thank you, I've decided to go to Selfridges, they can teach me more, I do hope you still have time to reach the other people you interviewed and that you find someone satisfactory, I wouldn't like to feel I'd let you down, which impresses them. They wish her luck and tell her to come back if she ever wants to change jobs. I'm thrilled with the way Vicki has handled all this – it's a tremendous boost to her ego too – she and I bounce! She tries to phone George but he isn't there. She fetches Martin to help her work on the old bike – they spend all evening on it, in the hall, as I reckon they'll make a better job of it in the warm.

At 10:30 p.m. George appears.

There is an article in the paper today about removing bone marrow, cleaning it by sticking polystyrene beads to it and passing it over a magnet, freezing it, then returning it to the patient. In this country.

George doesn't want to know. Anything. He asks about our week but as usual doesn't want to hear the word 'blood' mentioned. It's practically impossible to discuss either our week or leukaemia without mentioning blood. And it must not become an unmentionable word in this house.

He hides behind a newspaper, nothing to report to us, not wanting to hear our news. I retire to bed and leave him there.

He is not part of the family, he's a draining occasional presence and brings tension into the house. We're all rather nervous of him. It's so sad, and I don't know how it's happened. Don't sleep.

Saturday 14 January

Wake George with tea at 9:00. He complains Cat woke him at 4:00 – rush to check Cat, who's still in one piece and looks unruffled.

George takes Vicki into Thame to buy various bits for her bike, shoes and a dark sweater for her job; they come home without shoes or sweater, both extremely touchy. While George sleeps after lunch I work hard to get Vicki into a love-your-father frame of mind, explaining that he's over-tired, over-worked and probably just plain scared at the thought of flying to New York tomorrow in this terrible gale; we can all be touchy without meaning to upset people when we're under stress. Later remind George the turbulence must be very close to the ground, he'll soon be up and above it.

He leaves me a couple of phone numbers, New York and Melbourne, but no dates or schedule or flight numbers as he usually does. Puzzling. I think he feels bad about going so far away just now. He says if I want him he'll return immediately; I reckon my chances of locating him in an emergency are more remote than ever before. Don't even know how to reach him in London as he hasn't given me his new address or phone number. He says he'll phone me every three or four days.

Grandad didn't feel well enough to come to lunch today. His legs are very bad and he says he has such lumps he can't even get his socks on, the doctor is coming and he thinks he'll have to go into hospital again.

Justin's auntie phones and offers to collect Vicki tomorrow and take her back to school with Justin. Discover Vicki hasn't yet told Justin that she has left school and is only going back to collect a few things, see him and return on Monday.

Adam spends most of the day lying on the rug in front of the fire, surrounded by cushions. Coughs, doesn't want food but drinks plenty of water.

Ain't life great.

Sunday 15 January
Frantic early-morning clearing up activity – thank heavens – Justin's auntie looks like Zsa Zsa Gabor but with perhaps more make-up and jewellery adorning her. She's pleasant though.

Adam dresses today. Quiet, tearful, still coughing.

Monday 16 January
Windy and raining. Suggest we go and see poor Grandad, and Adam swallows his medicine very quickly, dresses. Grandad pleased to see us, recounts how he put his cigarette down, left the room, returned to find the waste-paper basket on fire, burnt the taps when he put it into the washbasin and then hurt his knees cleaning up the mess. Has a lump on his thigh as well as swollen ankles and is very frightened of the possibility of another operation. Try to cheer him up, praise his initiative in dealing with the fire, recommend not leaving cigarettes unattended, reassure him about the cost of new taps and about lumpy legs, hug and kiss him and promise we'll come again soon.

Adam and I buy Vicki an alarm clock like his and then collect her from the station. She's very touchy. Announces she's going up to school every other weekend, that she'll get another job which pays more, that in the summer she's going to work for Justin's father in Australia. I expect she's a little nervous about tomorrow. I let it all swim over me; now is not the time to debate all that.

Tuesday 17 January
Get up at 7:00 to have coffee with Vicki before she sets off. When I wave her goodbye at 7:20 in the cold and dark, I feel as I did when I first left her at school when she was four . . . She's just as vulnerable in her way, it's going to seem just as long a day, everyone and everything new. At least the gale has dropped, I don't have to worry she'll be blown off her bike on her way to the bus.

Fairly quick Clinic today, Drs Evelyn, Morrison, and Keith all there. Adam's blood all right.

I ask what they can tell me about monoclonal antibodies and polystyrene beads. Someone from haematology acknowledges I'd asked something along those lines last week and said that although the system may prove in the future to be relevant, right now it isn't, as the haematological antibodies all have things in common which means that leukaemic cells cannot be separated from ordinary cells, more particularly the stem cells which are about-to-divide blood cells, and therefore cannot be killed off without also disposing of necessary cells. In the case quoted in the papers, although the cancer was *in* the bone marrow, it wasn't *of* the bone marrow; the process unfortunately isn't applicable in our case. At least I think that's what he said.

Dr Morrison sends Adam out of the room with a nurse and asks me if he's still depressed and would I like to see the child psychologist. Say I don't think he is depressed – he feels low as a result of medication, radiotherapy, being anaemic. Agreed. Asks, Is he back at school yet? I say, No, he isn't nearly ready and quite honestly they don't want the responsibility; explain that to my mind in Adam's case little stimulating excursions more beneficial to him than formal schooling anyway, explain one or two things I have in mind for when he's strong enough. Dr Morrison agrees I could continue like that for the time being, says that I appear to be approaching the problem in an intelligent manner. Gee thanks.

We visit Willow's puppies, and later I phone Phil to see if he thinks it would be all right for me to phone Thame Police Station to ask if I could take Adam on a visit there. Phil says he doesn't think Thame is big enough to be very interesting and immediately offers to fetch Adam himself one day next week and take him to the Police Headquarters at Kidlington, show him the cells, handcuffs, police cars. I'm terribly touched by his kindness – hadn't meant to trouble him at all.

Vicki returns at 6:30. I needn't have worried, she's had a very exciting and stimulating day. There was a fire practice – Madam, that is the fire alarm, *please* stop trying things on and come out now; a stolen credit card showed up on her till code system – Oh dear, I'm so sorry, I've pressed the wrong button, would you mind waiting while I fetch my supervisor. She likes the people she's working with, and has a theatre date for Thursday. The front of a nearby shop collapsed onto the pavement, injuring people. This is *life*.

9

Wednesday 18 January
I suggest to Adam that we go and explore the Pitt Rivers Museum, which both Briony and Willow think he would enjoy, and he swallows his medicine down and dresses, quite enthusiastic.

We look round the University Museum as the Pitt Rivers part doesn't open till 2:00; see some impressive-looking animal skeletons, a collection of rather moth-eaten stuffed birds, some lovely beetles, butterflies and crystals. Adam interested, then when he says he's hungry we go to a restaurant but once inside he's not hungry, he wants to come home. In the street he turns very white, faint and unbalanced – have to hold him up, put him into a taxi to get him back to my car where he immediately falls asleep. I'm so glad the taxi-driver accepted us – he could so easily have thought, This looks like trouble; no. You brush against the nicest people when you're most in need of them.

Once home, Adam doesn't stir from the sofa all afternoon, sleeps most of the time. Do favourite baked stuffed potatoes with tomato and cucumber salad for supper but he says, No, he's off food. Vicki goes out when she's had hers.

Thursday 19 January
Sunny, frosty, no wind for once. Vicki goes off on the bus which she has just discovered runs from the village, will be brought back from the theatre this evening.

Adam white, silent, flat out on the sofa in his pyjamas and dressing-gown, cuddling Cat. Can't get him doing anything, but I can make him smile.

I ask a farmer if there is any early lambing around here, he'd enjoy stroking baby lambs. Have a wild idea that if there's an orphaned one we may be able to adopt and bottle-feed it – surely that would be interesting enough to get him onto his feet.

Can't interest him in writing in his diary, writing to his teacher or even seeing how his cress is growing. Just being there quietly with him seems to comfort him. He wants to stay on the sofa all night. Tell him firmly that he'll be far more comfortable in bed, it'll get cold down here when the heating goes off in the night; he must brush his teeth anyway. He's determined not to brush his teeth and shows more spirit about this than anything else during the last 24 hours.

I wonder why I'm resenting George's attitude so much. Events over the past few months substantiate his non-participation in family life; why is it now more difficult for me to live with? Even he can't feel he's contributing much. I don't feel I'm giving him anything either. I wish we could help each other. I'm grateful that he keeps coming back; he must feel as uneasy as I do.

Friday 20 January

By 10.45 I've persuaded Adam to get dressed. We go first to collect his septrin prescription and see Nick, so I ask him what a doctor understands by depression, in case Dr Morrison was right. Nicholas thinks after discussion that my interpretation is right; I'm relieved not to have to start taking him to a child psychologist. Nick thinks it may be helpful to contact the Helen House Hospice; he'll sound them out on my behalf and pop round some time next week.

Adam and I shop, have toasted cheese sandwiches and salad for lunch then decide it's a lovely day for a bonfire. There's a certain exhilaration about a fire. The Vicar calls and enjoys it with us for a little while – Adam and me, one Old English Sheepdog, one cat, four bantams and eleven ducks. And Horace.

It's Vicki's late evening, a man follows her from the bus in the dark and frightens her. Cuddles, hot sweet tea, calm her down. She won't hear of my telling Phil.

Grandad rings. He doesn't feel well, his legs are swollen, he has phlebitis, and could I fetch him over for lunch tomorrow. I'll have to find out what phlebitis is, and make sure Adam can't catch it.

Saturday 21 January

Phlebitis is something to do with his varicose veins. Adam has a pyjamas and dressing-gown day after yesterday's activities. Collect Grandad – he was waiting for me at the door even though I arrived early. He seems pretty agile, although as usual his legs are such agony, Katherine, he doesn't know what he's going to do. Poor devil. He's on maximum analgesics.

It's frosty cold so I light a fire and we all spend the afternoon drowsing in front of it, then I take him back in time for his supper there. Drive down to the bus stop to make sure Vicki isn't followed; all is well and my concern pleases her. Point out safe houses. Loaf around reading to Adam, watching television with him, make supper.

George phones from Melbourne. Phil called earlier to say he'll collect Adam about 10:30 Wednesday to take him round the police headquarters – Adam is thrilled and tells George all about it.

Vicki has her supper and goes straight out. I'll have to ask her to tell her friends not to phone after 10:00 – Adam and I are disturbed by two phone calls after 11:00 tonight. An anti-social hour for a social call, in my mind.

Sunday 22 January
Lie in bed idly trying to guess the time from the light. Decide 7:45, but it's 9:15 and Adam comes in with coffee for me, bless him.

Vicki seems very low, Adam has no breakfast, no lunch; plays Donkey Kong all day, gets furious with it, curses loudly when he misses.

However can I get this family going again?

Weigh Adam after his bath: 7st. 10lb. and he's as tall as me.

Monday 23 January
Adam has a very good day. We do the chores together this morning; play I-Spy while I'm working in the kitchen. He wins: he spied something beginning with 'U' which I simply couldn't guess: onion. Of course. I should have known!

Help him write another letter to his teacher, then we go to lunch with Ben and Jane. Soup, spaghetti and cider in the kitchen. Ben and Jane are so kind, and it's delightful. Adam begins to keel over around 2:30 so we come home and light a fire.

Angela arrives during the evening; it's very good to see her, and we talk till late.

Tuesday 24 January

Reasonably quick Clinic. Adam's blood count is up a little so the medication is increased to half maximum. Maximum dose of drugs is calculated (on the square meterage of the child) to reduce the number of white cells to around 1,000 per cubic millimetre of blood. Below this level natural resistance to infection is decreased to a dangerous level, so the drugs are stopped or decreased as appropriate to allow the white cell count to creep up again. Platelet level is checked, and so is haemoglobin in case of anaemia. I begin to appreciate the importance of blood tests and marvel at the speed with which the path. lab. sends all this vital information down to the doctors. Adam's very excited about tomorrow – I do hope there won't be a police emergency which would mean Phil's putting him off.

Vicki returns looking fresh, pretty, friendly and bubbly. I tell her the first part of the compatibility test looks okay and they want her to come along with us next Tuesday to give a blood sample for the following phase of the testing. She doesn't seem to mind, cheerfully goes up for a bath. Adam takes a letter from Justin up to her, and when she comes down she's surly and uptight again but won't say what, if anything, is the matter. She goes off to Youth Club with Martin and without supper. Adam doesn't want any supper, either; Angela and I eat alone. She plays a lot with Adam and he responds beautifully. It's good for him to have the stimulation of someone other than me.

Wednesday 25 January

Today sparkles with sunny frost and Adam sparkles too as he walks up to the orchard in his moonboots to feed the ducks. He's been ready for ages, washed, teeth brushed, in his anorak and woolly hat, waiting for Phil. Angela says she's never seen such excitement, how can he contain it?

While he's out Angela and I walk Sheba through the fields and talk a lot. Adam is back by 2:30, happy but very tired. He had sausages and chips for lunch in the police canteen, saw the workshop where they maintain the police vehicles, had his photo taken wearing a sergeant's jacket and cap. They took him for a burn-up on the motorway in a 'jam sandwich' and let Adam work the siren. He was given several fact-sheets about police work and history, and a shield to hang on his wall which Phil says is only given to Very Special Visitors. He tells us all this between little dozes on the sofa, and holds his shield and the leaflets very tightly all evening. This has given him so much pleasure, I wish I could adequately express my gratitude to Phil.

Thursday 26 January
Angela and I clean a few things then get Adam dressed and go to visit Grandad. Adam takes his police things to show him. Grandad rather more muddled than usual but cheerful. Angela, Adam and I then have a very good pub lunch in Long Crendon, come home and spend a hilarious afternoon on the floor playing jumping frogs and other daft games.

Angela makes haggis and neeps for supper (Burns Night), it's a new experience for me. We drink whisky which she says is essential and talk late.

Friday 27 January
Drizzling but warmer and the birds are vocal in their appreciation. Angela zooms round with the vacuum cleaner, washes the kitchen floor – says she came to be useful – then kisses us goodbye. We send love to her family, thanks for sparing her.

Adam white and won't dress. Tuck him up in his rug on the sofa with Cat, rush off to the shop and when I get back he's dressed, wandering round the garden! We take Sheba for a walk and he brings his binoculars in case we see the white-tailed eagle which is living around here just now. An eight foot wing span – even I should be able to recognise it! From Draycott to Brill the place is crawling with ornithologists, it's the first time in 90 years this bird has been seen in this country. Poor lost thing. We see nothing larger than crows. Rooks. (If you see one rook, it's a crow; several crows are rooks.)

Adam goes next door to show off his police things and tell them about his trip. Nick Peters calls, says the Helen House people are not appropriate just now. He chats for a while, and to Adam when he comes in; seems satisfied with us. I think.

Help Adam to shave round his chin and upper lip after his bath. This is his first shave and he appreciates the dignity of the occasion. Tells me he might try drinking beer when he's a bit older, and goes to bed, happy, with Cat.

Saturday 28 January
After driving Vicki to the station so she could go to school for the weekend, Adam and I set off to try to find the sea eagle. All the lanes to Long Crendon and Brill are lined with cars, ornithologists in dun and green with telescopes on tripods litter the verges. On the Brill/Crendon road they tell us it went to ground after eating a rabbit (quite a change after fish I should think) and that it's definitely adult but they don't know whether it's male or female (if it's that adaptable, I should think female). Visit Brill windmill as a small diversion – find it this time – drive around some more. Wherever we go they lost sight of it two minutes before. At Long Crendon we are reliably informed it's definitely a juvenile . . . I'm quite interested in the ornithologists as a species; they are very friendly and remarkably similar, but Adam becomes impatient to go home.

Sunday 29 January
Mild and sunny. Adam plays outside with Lennie for a couple of hours then comes with me to fetch Grandad.

He's very spry, swollen ankles and phlebitis both gone, but is still full of petty complaints. Tucks into a hearty lunch. I think probably he needs to eat so much because his digestive system is no longer able to extract as much nourishment from his food as it should, so he needs an ever-increasing volume to compensate. Another of my theories . . .

Adam and Grandad loaf in front of the fire and I walk Sheba round the fields, wondering how I can feel almost happy, out in the open countryside. Incongruous, in the circumstances.

Conversation with Adam about hand-washing. No, of course your willy isn't dirty, no way, and any germs in your pee are yours and okay thank you. But lavatories are used by several people in between being cleaned and someone else's germs may not be so friendly. Yes you do have to touch the lavatory: I like gentlemen to lift the seat before they use it, I like the seat and the lid lowered again afterwards – for one thing, it prevents Sheba stopping by for a quick drink – and furthermore I like the lavatory to be flushed after use; so much nicer for the next person along. So, it's sensible then to wash one's hands. *Both* hands, my friend, even if you do manage with one hand . . .

Adam writes a nice thank-you letter to Phil; we collect Vicki who has had a very good weekend with all her friends.

Monday 30 January
Deliver thank-you letters to Phil, flowers to Granny's grave and call on Mandy for eggs. She hauls us in to see three new calves, one home produced, two bought-in Charolais; lovely, Adam and I both enjoy seeing them. Buying eggs from Mandy invariably offers more than just free-range eggs; there is usually a new-born something which it delights her to show off as much as it does us to see and stroke.

Adam has adopted a new swear word. When he's mad at Donkey Kong or at me, he'll say, Oh . . . *Radish*! It's a distinct improvement on the words he learnt at school, and you can get a lot of invective into it. I plan to use it myself.

Victoria says the nurse in Selfridges says she drinks far too much and while they're at it tomorrow could they also test her for diabetes. Oh, please God, no . . .

Tuesday 31 January
Vicki okay, Maxine says no sign of sugar in urine. It's probably hot and dry in Selfridges.

Adam has vincristine as well as blood sample taken and is so scared all his veins disappear. Dr Keith has three shots, the haematologist manages it in the end. Adam is flat out and sobbing even when Maxine makes Dr Keith cough up 20p for dud attempts. Adam's blood count is 968 which is low. The pharmacy don't have enough mercaptopurine or prednisone, phone other Oxford hospitals which don't have any either. Wait another hour or so, and am then told Maxine will bring further supplies out to us on Thursday.

Adam screams, thumps me, spits, twists my fingers while I try to give him his medicine tonight. I'm at my wits' end – we can't spill this – wondering whether I should bring in reinforcements in the shape of Willow or Chris, Briony or Ted, but I can't expect them to supervise his medicine twice daily, we must work it out for ourselves. We both dissolve into exhausted tears, hug each other and he takes it, without spilling any; we're friends again before bathtime.

I'm devastated, at 4:00 still shaking and too tense to sleep.

Wednesday 1 February
Another pyjamas and dressing-gown day, and the prednisone certainly hasn't increased his appetite yet.

His teacher, Mrs Wolf, comes to tea. We have egg sandwiches with Adam's homegrown cress. She brought him a tape which the school had made, and has a connection who could arrange a visit to a fire station for us – super! She asks Adam to write to her again – she's great. He loves the tape, plays it over and over again.

Thursday 2 February
Still not wanting to dress, my son swears Radish at video games while I do some household jobs. Maxine visits with further drug supplies, says we aren't allowed use of the pool at the orthopaedic hospital (extra warm) – it was worth asking though, he loves swimming and an ordinary pool would be too cold for him just now. She says it seems older children do take longer to get over things, but as each one reacts differently she can't give me any idea of how long it'll be before he's something like normal again.

George phones. He's back, he's tired, he's been in meetings all day, he doesn't know when he'll have time to come back here – *and*, in Australia they can cure T-cell leukaemia, no problem.

Friday 3 February
Bitter wind, Adam's wise to stay out of it. His headteacher has set the wheels in motion for a home tutor. George phones to say he'll be back sometime tomorrow after looking at a house in St John's Wood. Adam can't make up his mind whether or not he'd like to go out to lunch tomorrow; says he may just want to sleep on his bed.

Saturday 4 February
Take Vicki to the station for the early train again. George arrives midday and we take Adam out to a restaurant for lunch – he tucks well into avocado and pheasant.

This evening when Adam's in bed George tries to explain to me about the new cure for T-cell leukaemia his Australian friend told him about. Apparently two drug companies and a university in the USA have been genetic engineering together, and discovered drugs which will cure AIDS and T-cell leukaemia. They are, it seems, simply awaiting drug licences before releasing this knowledge to the world and making their fortunes. Because it involves changing the DNA, it will incur moral censure. I ask if disease doesn't change the DNA. Given that this information is correct, it'll probably take six to ten years to filter through, I reckon.

I wish I could believe in fairies.

Sunday 5 February
George and Adam study a boating catalogue, plan an Easter boating trip on the Avon and Severn ring – Adam is very excited. He's thrilled also with the walkabout radio/cassette and headphones which George brought him – ideal to take on a boat!

George goes off to fetch his father over for lunch, Adam watches me make pancakes. Sees his drugs, says, Good, my tablets are nearly gone. I say, Yes, but they'll give us more on Tuesday, tablets are now a part of life, my love. Adam says, This (the septrin) is good for me, but the tablets are poison and I'm going to die. Hug him and say, Oh you aren't going to die for a long time yet. Looking straight into my eyes he says, I am, you know: if I were in water and didn't swim I'd drown, wouldn't I. Then he makes a joke and goes away, leaving me icy cold, spoon in hand, mouth open, pancake burning.

Why doesn't he want to swim?

George has been a lot better this weekend, but there have been some bitter remarks about Vicki and Justin, their going to Australia plans. I ask him to be gentle with her, she's going to be disappointed in her dreams and plans anyway. Right, he says, I'll say nothing at all. Tell him that isn't what I want, either; he mutters about not being a good father and now it's too late. Say No, it can never be too late to show them that you love them and to encourage them. I thank him for the boating plans.

I wonder if he really wants out, or if he wants to be assured that he's needed.

10

Monday 6 February
Adam spends the day telling me he is *not* going to Clinic tomorrow, he *hates* giving blood. Nick calls and thinks he has a lot more bounce than last week – he's certainly a lot more bloody-minded!

Tuesday 7 February
Please God, bless Phil! He called this morning with photos of Adam in police uniform and in the police car – they're terrific, he looks as though he's been a police officer for years! Phil says not to tell Adam yet, but he's trying to get security clearance to take him to Upper Heyford to see the latest American jets. He'll take a day off work, collect Adam, an hour's drive there, a couple of hours looking around, an hour to get back – shouldn't be too tiring for him. Says he'd like to do that for Adam. It's so nice of him, it makes me cry.

It took a while to get Adam to Clinic this morning. I explain to Maxine that because of his bad experience last week he's dreading the blood sample, and could she show him what they do with it, to add a little interest. Joanne takes the blood – she's good at it, never has to take more than one shot – Adam hangs on to my hand and is brave. Then she and Maxine take him up to the lab. to see it going through the machine which counts white cells.

Dr Morrison tells us his blood is fine, up to ¾ treatment, come back in two weeks! Adam and I feel a Tuesday off is a bonus! Takes his medicine with no fuss this evening.

Vicki produces a college brochure from Justin's father; the interior design course she's interested in sounds very comprehensive, but it doesn't alter the fact that Australia is on the other side of the world, and I doubt she'd be eligible anyway.

Wednesday 7 February
Howling winds during the night bring down two of the ivy-covered plum trees in the hedge by the vegetable garden. No other damage, and electricity is still on.

Adam and I lunch with Thea, and stop en route to visit his old friends at Chiltern School.

Thursday 8 February
Adam has been having bad dreams recently. The only one he can tell me about concerns doctors who have a very fierce dog which they tell to bite and kill Adam. Put in a lot of propaganda for doctors. Ted and Briony most obligingly have a sweet elderly arthritic labrador; take Adam to buy a bone for her then we go and make friends.

Friday 9 February
Get through to Mrs Wolf's fireman friend and arrange to take Adam 10:00 on Sunday – he's delighted. It's so good for him to have something to look forward to. After lunch he sleeps on the sofa, seems off-colour; first his leg, then his shoulder, then his hand hurt. Normal quota of bacon sandwiches, sausages and chips disappear though.

After we've picked Vicki up Adam announces he's going to bed, but doesn't want to get undressed. Take his temperature: 101.5. Give him paracetamol. He throws up a couple of times. Call the duty doctor, who finds no indication of infection and phones the JR who say, Bring him in about 10:00 in the morning. Doctor says to give him more paracetamol in a while and plenty of fluids, take his temperature again in the morning, call him again if I'm worried in the night.

Saturday 10 February
Temperature just up – 100.4, so take him in. Examination, chest X-ray, show no reason for raised temperature. Blood sample taken and we return home at lunchtime with instructions to continue paracetamol to reduce temperature and to phone the doctor about 6:00 for blood test results and instructions re evening medication. George returns around 4:00. Take Adam's temperature just prior to ringing: 99.1, which is reassuring. The doctor says his blood count is 2.9 which is high, he'll get the differential and call me back. He

does so in a few minutes, says 2.9 is fine, the polymorphs are 60% (which is apparently good) and do continue medication at present level. I'm to bring Adam to Clinic on Tuesday, call if I'm worried before then, but if I bring him in again it'll mean admission.

The first time a blood count number is mentioned to me, it's 27, dangerously high. Next time, it's 968, too low. Now it's 2.9, high corrected to all right . . .?

Temperature up again at bedtime.

Sunday 11 February

Temperature 100.4 and Adam obviously unwell, but he's so keen on the Fire Station visit that George and I decide postponing it would create greater trauma than going, so I take him; George won't come. Very kind people, an interesting trip, but Adam too unwell to respond. They simulate an emergency call, dive into their waterproofs and boots and shoot off with sirens screaming, reappear and do drill with ladders and hoses. They let him climb all over their fantastic machines, explain things, give him a T-shirt, badges and a wall plaque. Can these people halfway imagine what their kindness means to a sick child?

George fetches his father over for lunch and I somehow manage to produce a proper roast lunch and pudding. Grandad keeps losing one of his sticks, which is an indication of greater mobility although he won't admit it . . .

George decides on a different boat trip, on the Thames, closer to the JR . . . Adam's temperature fluctuates.

Monday 13 February

A poor day, culminating again in a slight temperature.

Tuesday 14 February

Manage with difficulty to get Adam to Clinic. There's no accounting for his temperature. He gains tremendous comfort from Cat; spends most of the day curled up on the sofa with her.

Wednesday 15 February

A pyjamas and dressing-gown day. Freezing fog outside. Light the fire, Adam and Cat spend all day lying on the rug on cushions in front of it. Temperature below normal this evening. He eats one toasted sandwich, is reluctant to drink, says if he drinks he'll only have to get up and go to the loo. Cuddle him a lot, we read a little. He only really wants to stroke Cat and idly watch television. Hang up the bird-cake we made, he only watches the birds for a few minutes.

Thursday 16 February
Light fire and Adam moves downstairs with Cat. The Educational Psychologist calls and will recommend home tutoring for an hour a day (excluding Tuesdays) to start with. He tells me even if Adam doesn't do any work, talking to a teacher or even listening to a teacher talking to me would be beneficial to him, and offers to help in any way I might think would further stimulate him.

Maxine comes after lunch, says Dr Keith wants Adam back in for a while to try to find out what is causing his slightly raised temperature and obviously unwell feeling. Adam agrees. He has glasses of water, no food all day, goes to bed at 8:00.

Vicki comes home wanting to know if I've written to Justin's father yet about her going to Australia to college. No, I haven't, and I'm losing my cool again.

Friday 17 February
Adam is very tired from the effort involved in getting up to the Ward, leans on me while he sits in Sister's office as we wait for a room to be prepared.

Once again, they can find no reason for his raised temperature and ill feeling. He's examined thoroughly, urine sample, blood sample, chest X-ray.

George comes back and takes me to dinner with Duncan and Ruth. I'm glad to have the opportunity of a quiet word with Duncan, a paediatrician, who is supportive and sweet to me. We arrive home about 1:00 to discover neither of us has keys; throw stones at Victoria's window with eventual success.

Saturday 18 February
Adam waited for me to wash him. Still has a slight temperature but seems more responsive than he has been for days, which is nice for George.

I suggest when he's in Australia in April, could he call on Justin's parents? And my mother? He thinks he could do that.

Sunday 19 February
Adam asleep when I arrive at the JR, has a tablespoonful of lunch, sleeps again till 4:00. Temperature normal till he sits up and starts taking notice of things, then it goes back up again. He has half a cheese sandwich for supper, lies watching television. Misses Cat, sends me home at 6:45 to feed her. Duncan's hospital has rabbits, why can't Cat come to our hospital?

Vicki returns by taxi after a good weekend with her friends.

Monday 20 February
Adam in better spirits, eats a fish finger for lunch. Watches television all morning, sleeps all afternoon, has half a hamburger and three baked beans for supper – things are looking up! Vicki comes in to see him after work and I take her home with me. She's tired after a busy weekend.

Tuesday 21 February
Adam sitting up watching television when I arrive. See Dr Morrison and ask if he could speed up the compatibility testing, explain that Vicki wants to go abroad.

Have a useful talk in the parents' sitting room with Doreen, little Joe's mother. He's in with an infection she hopes he will throw off quickly as he's due to go in to the Westminster for his transplant next week – he's T-cell too. She says T-cell cancer is likely to come back in spite of transplantation, also the risk of infection is so great that they were instructed at the Westminster to get rid of the family pets and not to keep any animals for at least a year afterwards.

Debbie is back in with little Kirsty, whose heart rhythms are becoming very difficult to regulate and they're changing her drugs. Debbie is hopeful that Magdi Yacoub will look at Kirsty's papers; the position has been explained to him and he thinks he may be able to remove the tumour.

Wednesday 22 February
Home again, I offer Adam consommé or scrambled egg but he decides he just wants a little plain boiled brown rice. I suppose his instinct tells him what is acceptable after more than

a week of near-starvation. He eats about a dessertspoonful.

Justin has apparently been sent down from school for being some place he shouldn't have been; Victoria wants me to have him live here. I've said no, but he can stay at weekends when she'll be around to keep him company. She says he'd pay me £20 a week for his keep so it'd be all right, wouldn't it? Say no again, it isn't that, I'm not running a boarding house, it's that I have rather a lot on my plate at the moment and I just don't need anyone else to think about, to feed, to drive around.

Vicki starts sobbing that people at work have told her that the bone marrow thing was extremely painful and that she'd be left badly scarred; she didn't even like giving blood samples and she's frightened. Try to allay her fears. Nothing would ever be done without full explanation and consent from her; I wouldn't ask anything of her for Adam that I wouldn't ask of him for her; the whole thing is fairly unlikely anyway but if it were possible it'd be done under general anaesthetic, they'd make sure she had no pain, and as she wouldn't be cut she couldn't be scarred. Appreciate that she would like Justin's support but I simply can't take on anything else just now. I'm sorry if Justin has alienated both school and his grandparents, but that is his problem, not mine.

Feel terrible, sure I haven't dealt with this in the right way.

Thursday 23 February

Adam feels cold and spends the day in front of the fire with Cat. Looks beautiful, vulnerable, shudders at the suggestion of food. Sips water if I make him. I feel high on anxiety, twisting snakes in my stomach, unreliable knees. Must *make* myself strong. The iron hand in the oven glove?

Adam consents to a half-hearted game of jumping frogs which makes him laugh. This evening he asks for two boiled eggs and toast soldiers – rush through to do them – he manages most of one egg and one soldier, decides to have a bath and go to bed. Weighs 7st. He's lost 10lb. in ten days, no wonder he feels cold and lacking in energy.

On the news I hear a 12-year-old boy with immune deficiency disease who has lived his life in a sterile bubble has died after a bone marrow transplant from his sister.

Friday 24 February
Dive into Thame to do a quick shop and some lunatic traps me in the car park. It's half an hour before I can get out and I'm in an absolute panic. Adam of course is quite all right. I'm carrying more logs in when Nick arrives – he tells Adam he must eat to get strong again. He called at the hospital, spoke to the doctors, says Adam is over his infection now. I ask if he considers animals a source of infection and he evades neatly. Seems to watch me closely, says he'll call in again next week.

Decide eating is more fun in company and invite Chris and Willow to supper on Monday. Go over to see Ted, who says firmly that our animals are necessary to our quality of life. He says I'm putting so much into all this, have I thought what I'll do if Adam doesn't come through it. Can't consider this. He says he's sure Adam isn't in any pain, none of them would let him be, and that I'm having the pain for him. I'll try to believe that. He is a beautiful man. He tries again to make me cry, hugs me.

Saturday 25 February
Adam just lies on the sofa wrapped in his rug. George appears at 1:30, has lunch, disappears to shop and visit his father, reappears at 6:30 and spends the evening house-hunting in the newspapers.

Sunday 26 February
It's 10:30 and I've already lit the fire, done the animal chores, when first Adam then George appear downstairs – Adam dressed, George in pyjamas! Adam asks for a fluffy milkshake for breakfast then can't drink it. George complains that (a) I haven't yet completed the parochial church register return; (b) I hadn't attended meeting re proposed building near village hall; (c) part of his trellis blew down in the gale and (d) he can't find a converter to plug his hair-drier into – neither Vicki's hair-drier nor mine will do. I almost burst, but he goes off to fetch his father just in time.

Adam joins us at the lunchtable, eats about a tablespoonful and is sick, retires to rest in front of the fire again.

Collect Vicki from the station this evening and the first thing she says is, Have you collected my bracelet from the mender's?

I just don't seem able to do half the things people expect of me.

Adam manages to keep down a cup of tomato soup, goes to bed halfway through watching a film on television.

There seems to be a sort of domino effect in life: when one structure collapses the adjacent ones go down too, one after the other. Hold onto the fact that, after the second worst week in my life, Adam is still here – and so am I! It feels amazing.

11

Monday 27 February
Adam can't drink his soup at lunchtime, rests after the attempt. Willow and Chris are lovely supper guests, no hassle, and Adam eats!

Victoria's visa application and information from Australia House arrive; she's very pleased.

Tuesday 28 February
Adam has a milkshake and some sponge fingers before going to Clinic. Dr Evelyn says so far his blood and Vicki's are identical, so we'll go on to the stage 3 testing. If that goes well we should seriously consider transplantation, and did I realise a second course of radiation would leave Adam slightly more retarded. No.

He says I'm to get Adam eating more and outside playing football, but doesn't suggest how!

Adam eats lunch, sleeps all afternoon, has a light supper and goes to bed early.

Vicki is upset to hear another blood sample required.

Wednesday 29 February
Vicki goes to the dentist, Emma comes to lunch. Adam is very pleased to see her and he eats a whole steak, potatoes, mushrooms, beans but no salad, then raspberries and kiwi fruit! Don't know about him, but it does me a power of good! Vicki appears with two fillings and finishes the fruit. Nick calls in this evening, pleased to see Adam brighter and hear he's eating better; he'll come to lunch with us on Thursday. He's so nice, and it does help Adam to see a doctor on a social occasion rather than just on business. He still has nightmares about them.

He bathes early, weighs 6st. 12 lb. . . .

Thursday 1 March
Always glad to see the back of February, and today is mild and sunny, the crocuses have their star faces smiling open. Adam manages his medicine, dresses and comes with me to Viv's to have my hair done. I hate having my hair done. But the operation is very much more pleasant when all I have to do is stroll down to the other end of the village and sit in Viv's comfortable kitchen, chat to her while she does her bit and Adam watches television.

Adam comes shopping with me, leans on the trolley in the supermarket so heavily I'm afraid he's going to pass out, but we manage to get back to the car. On our return, Little Black Bantam makes her Look at me – I've laid an egg! cry, from the top of the willow tree. We can't see if she really has.

George phones to say he's arranged to take Adam on a longboat on Saturday *if* it's fine, Adam's well enough, etc. He'll collect him on Saturday morning. Great.

Leave Victoria in charge of Adam this evening while I go to the leukaemia Clinic parents' evening. A haematologist gives a talk. I'd misunderstood the rejection point in transplantation – it's the new bone marrow, of course, which tries to reject the recipient's body, not the other way round. I should have realised, if I'd really thought about it.

The operation has a 50% chance of success, it's two or three weeks of isolation afterwards and not as long before as I had thought, Tuesday to Saturday usually. As well as lowering the IQ, the second dose of radiation – six hours, which is an essential preliminary to transplantation and about which no one knows the long-term effects – has the effect of sterilising boys. There is the possibility of cataracts; the terrifying solitude of the aftermath of the operation itself, and the possibility of graft-versus-host disease to some degree; the dreaded pneumono-something; the possibility of tight skin, which apparently is a condition leaving the patient with permanently painful and almost immobile hands. A certain percentage relapse late after transplantation, so one can't count them as cured till three to five years after the operation. Girls have a better chance than boys.

As Vicki and Adam so far have identical blood – there are four antigens they can identify, numerous others they can't type – they will go ahead with the next part of the testing,

HLA I think he said, mixing lymphocytes from both of them to see how compatible they are.

I asked, I understood one gets a disease through a genetic susceptibility which was triggered by some outside factor, e.g. a virus. Therefore, if they put in fresh but identical bone marrow, for example from an identical twin, without locating and removing the trigger, weren't you simply back at square one? Not answered.

He said most of our children were on 50%–75% maintenance treatment, they liked to have them as high as their tolerance would allow. Adam is tolerating well just now, on maximum. If this is tolerating well, I think I want to keep him on chemotherapy rather than try anything more drastic.

I ask what transplantation is like for the donor. He says they take a pint of blood a couple of weeks before, then on T-day they anaesthetise the donor, make 6–8 punctures in the skin around the pelvic girdle and, because the skin is flexible, that allows them to syphon off around 500 ml. blood and bone marrow from various places through these punctures. Previously-collected blood is then returned to the donor, who is very sore for a couple of days and most sympathetically treated with painkillers, even heroin. And no, no one had come back for more heroin.

A most informative evening, I have plenty to get my teeth into.

Get home at 11:00 to find Adam waiting for me to do his hot-water bottle and hear his prayers, kiss him goodnight. My poor Adam, I love you so much.

Friday 2 March
Maxine rings and tells me to bring them both to 4B on Tuesday for blood samples.

Saturday 3 March
Vicki off for the weekend again; Adam packed, ready and excited by the time George comes for him at 10:00. Send Adam on a final tour of the house to make sure he hasn't forgotten anything, and to give me a chance to tell George that the first two blood tests are compatible. No response. Tell him that the parents' meeting on Thursday was most informative and interesting, it's a pity he couldn't come. No response. Then he

bursts out that he can't understand the instructions on this roll of film, *where* are the camera instructions?

Why doesn't he want to know?

Sunday 4 March

Go to early service, comb and trim Sheba, sleep, comb and trim Sheba. George tired and snappy when he brings Adam home; Adam blooming, pink and interested – he's had a super time and the floor is still going up and down.

Monday 5 March

Adam sleeps most of the day. The bantam *is* nesting on top of the willow tree, of course we have to have chickens of an independent nature! Toy with the idea of taking Adam to Bournemouth for a few days, I think the break and the sea air would do us both good. I'm feeling odd and disorientated too. Vicki says she'll manage but we haven't gone into detail.

We have supper with Willow and Chris; Willow helps Adam make a little pink pig out of folded paper. We enjoy ourselves. Adam eats well but tires early in spite of all the sleep he's had today.

Tuesday 6 March

Take Adam and Vicki to 4B, Vicki well-doped with Valium. She had to have two blood samples taken because Dr Keith did the wrong thing with the first one. She cleans her room furiously for the rest of the day, is very scratchy and uptight, poor love, doesn't relax till evening.

Adam is hungry and he writes a nice thank-you letter for the hospitality he received on the boat. Laughs himself silly over finding some ancient false teeth under the hedge, wants to know if Grandad sneezed them out while last getting into the car! Grandad's girl-friend Edith has had a stroke, we must see him tomorrow.

Victoria on the phone to Justin for half an hour. They write daily, too. I wish she had a burning ambition, a vocation. I wish I didn't envisage my daughter marrying young, divorcing, remarrying, finding herself in 15 years' time standing in the middle of a supermarket somewhere, surrounded by children and wondering how she got there and who she is. Sex is super but there are other important things in life.

Wednesday 7 March
Get up at 4:15, certain I can hear someone moving about downstairs. There's no one, of course, but I get going.

Visit Grandad, who has apparently been driving everyone mad about money recently. He wrote a cheque for £100 without naming a payee: they tore it up. Edith still needs a lot of rest which is difficult for him to understand. He wants to get her up and doing, wants money to take her out, although neither of them can move far without help. Poor Grandad.

Now Vicki is feeling neglected. She says no one has ever done anything for *her*, she was just pushed off to boarding school out of the way. Point out that she begged to go to boarding school. I wanted to keep my daughter at home, but as she wanted to go so badly we came around to the view that it would at least give her some freedom from the restrictions which life with Adam seemed to impose, give her an independence I consider invaluable. She won't accept it. Work hard trying to re-establish confidence, make her feel appreciated; how I enjoy her company but don't want to be selfish about it, still want her to be independent, to have her own life; Adam's problems demand priority but I try very hard not to let them restrict her too much, what else would she have me do, I'm open to suggestion. And I'm extremely grateful for her co-operation regarding blood samples, which I know is difficult for her.

Thursday 8 March
Adam comes in with four bantam eggs as well as two duck eggs, which he puts into a box for Dr Nicholas.

I'm too tense when he comes to make the most of it – I almost shoot the lamb on to the floor when I try to cut it, and the wine is appalling. He's so kind I feel I should – and could – really talk to him. Adam eats well but is unresponsive. Nick keeps saying, What a nice lunch, as though he'd expected a couple of lightly poached Valium with a whisky chaser. I didn't feel it was an unmitigated success.

Vicki isn't around much but makes a point of thanking me for the various sandwich fillings I've bought her. Think we are friends again – certainly hope so. This tightrope is difficult.

Saturday 10 March
I'm 45 today. Vicki gives me a nice card and some pinking shears which she knew I wanted, and helps Adam write a card for me before she goes off for the weekend.

George comes back at lunchtime, gives me a cheque for £1,000. Feel I'm being bought, somehow. He says it's so I can take Adam away, as well as buy myself something. I feel stupidly ungrateful; it's very nice of him and what on earth do I want? Perhaps someone to tell me I'm doing all right and cuddle me when things feel worst.

Tell George that the more I hear about transplantation the less I like the idea, and he *agrees*.

Sunday 11 March
Adam and I leave George poring over the property pages of the *Sunday Times* while we walk Sheba – it's a beautiful mild sunny day with spring in the air.

We all go to collect Grandad and take him out to lunch in Long Crendon to celebrate my birthday. Indifferent lunch but a pleasant outing – and it's nice to eat something I haven't had to think about, buy, bring home and peel, cook and serve. Grandad wants to go straight back after lunch to see how poor Edith is, and gives me a piece of paper I think may be birthday wishes, but it's a request to buy him one shirt and a pair of pyjamas. He eats so much he's bursting out of his clothes.

George leaves about 5:00 and Phil calls to say probably Wednesday for Upper Heyford – Adam ecstatic.

Monday 12 March
Letter telling me a Mr Dinton will be Adam's home tutor – expect to hear from him soon. Adam is pleased it'll be a man. Take Adam into Oxford, where we see Vicki at work, take her out to lunch, then buy Grandad his new shirt and pyjamas.

Vicki nearly has hysterics when I call her Victoria in Selfridges. She says she can't stand her name. Vicki is bad enough but Victoria is too unbearably snobby and she hates it. Did I ever do anything right?

Tuesday 13 March
Joanne takes blood sample while Adam holds tight onto my hand, then two fat tears slide down his cheeks. Joanne talks

on about chickens, her doves and dogs until he feels better; we both pretend not to notice the tears.

Dr Morrison says blood count is low so no treatment this week, just the septrin. He thinks it's a good idea to go to the seaside and, to my question about whether a vitamin supplement is indicated while Adam's appetite is so low, says no, most people have a sufficient supply to last years and folic acid is counter-indicated anyway, so a normal diet is okay. Say, But that's the point, he isn't having a normal diet, but he thinks it all right.

Home for a cup of consommé, then we take Grandad his new clothes, some cigarettes, sweets, matches.

12

Wednesday 14 March
Adam up and dressed early, nibbles some toast for breakfast. The sun shines through the mist and he's happy as he waits for Phil, who calls for him around 10:00, and brings Adam back about 2:30, stays for coffee. They saw the F1-11s, Adam climbed into the bomb space. He was shown missile launchers and given a ride in an armoured personnel vehicle (which he called a sweet little tank). They gave him a couple of polished-up nuclear-weapon cases, a T-shirt, a tie, two tie-pins, a very large photo of the fighter planes which they had all signed, various photos, leaflets and advertising stuff. He was thrilled with it all, gave Phil some eggs as a thank-you, won't let go of his stuff for long enough to write thank-you letters.

Thursday 15 March
Adam very excited at the prospect of going away, gets up and dresses early, does the animal chores for me; we post his thank-you letters, check tyres, fill up with petrol and set off before ten.

The driving is easy; we reach Bournemouth, also cold and grey, easily in two hours. Circle a little, looking at hotels, and decide on a three-star hotel just west of Exeter Road and the pier. They give us a nice little suite of main bedroom with easy chairs and television set, bathroom and small bedroom off. We have some lunch in the hotel, rest, then walk up the pier and watch the grey waves for a few minutes, walk back through the Gardens – the daffodils are in flower here, not yet at home. Rest in front of the television, then go down and play a wild game of table tennis for half an hour before having a drink and going in to dinner. Very civilised. Adam eats well, then we phone Vicki to let her know where we are – she has Sheba upstairs with her. Adam likes the hotel very much; I'm rather disappointed in the dining room.

Friday 16 March
Lovely sunny day, Adam slept well and wakens hungry. After breakfast we set off in the car to explore. All my childhood haunts have changed so much they're barely recognisable; only the sea and the swans are the same. And Bournemouth used to be so smart – we'd put on white gloves and Mother would wear a hat to go into town. Now it's scruffy with cardboard and polythene blowing about the gardens, so much building going on you feel you should walk about wearing a crash hat.

We return to rest. Later I persuade Adam down to dinner, he eats a little, doesn't look very well, leaves me to finish dinner by myself. The headwaiter insists on preparing a plate of biscuits and cheese for me to bring up in case Adam is hungry in the night, tells me the hall porter will provide sandwiches whenever he might want them. This from observation; nothing has been said. I'm melting again at the kindness of people. Go upstairs with a large Coke, the cheese and biscuits, a gin and tonic, to watch television with Adam.

Saturday 17 March
George phones while we're at breakfast; he's going to look at a couple of houses then go home to the village; wonder how he and Vicki will manage. Adam wants to stay in our suite watching Saturday-morning television so I go off around the shops.

Adam a little more lively on my return, so we set off in the car to Beaulieu. Gosh has Beaulieu changed! Last time I was there the motor museum was in a wooden shed, now it's all beautifully organised in lovely modern buildings. There's an information centre, a monorail, the fantastic collection of vintage cars and motor-bikes very well displayed. He enjoys it all, especially the monorail, but won't eat lunch. He likes good restaurants, not self-service cafeterias! Drive back through New Milton and Highcliffe, both unrecognisable. It doesn't do to go back to places twenty years and more after happy memories.

Sunday 18 March
Take Adam toast and marmalade upstairs. We drive round Poole Harbour looking at boats – and windsurfers who must

be frozen in spite of their wetsuits. Wonder if they're fur-lined for winter use. Walk across the sands a little way at Sandbanks, then return and Adam rests at the hotel while we wait for Pauline and John to come.

I take them all to the Carlton for lunch – it's a good lunch of course, and very good company too. Adam eats well and walks on the beach afterwards with John and Shandy while Pauline and I talk. Most emotive: haven't been back to the Carlton since our wedding reception.

I've had this car for more than a year now and still don't know how to unlock the petrol cap. At home it doesn't matter – I always use the local filling station and they know how to do it. Can't find a proper garage around here though. End up in one of those concrete deserts populated only by fourteen smug petrol pumps and one bored little girl in a glass cage. Turn the key this way and that, the petrol cap too, with no luck. It's like trying to get into Fort Knox. You'd think a handbook which illustrates and labels the steering wheel and gear lever for you could get around to letting you into the secret, wouldn't you. It doesn't. The first man I approach for help can't undo it either; the second does it easily, gives me a very strange look and actually *runs* back to his car. Incompetent I certainly am, but am I *that* scary?

Read the petrol pump and manage to fill the car, noticing towards the end of the operation that a hole in the sharp end of the pump is quietly directing a small but powerful jet of petrol down my trouser leg. Can't slot the damned thing back into its holder and *then* I can't make the petrol cap stay on. By this time I'm so flummoxed I try to pay the caged girl the number of litres rather than the price. Feel at any moment now she'll press a security button and kind men in white suits will arrive to take me away to a nice cosy padded cell. Drive off slowly with the windows open and hope you can't get high on petrol fumes.

Later, while rummaging in my bag for something, I notice all the vouchers for free glasses I've accumulated, wonder what the tax point is on petrol. If they *sold* you the glasses and *gave* you the petrol, would it still be taxable? Maybe I can get my own back. No, if it could work, someone would already have thought of it. Or they'd slap a 275% tax on glasses.

Monday 19 March

Home by lunchtime, but Adam doesn't want any. Cat and Sheba delighted to see us, Adam happy to be home with his animals. Phone his home tutor who comes to see us and will start on Wednesday.

Tuesday 20 March

Clinic. Dr Evelyn tells me I must forget the leukaemia and decide simply whether I want my child to live or die. On chemotherapy he has a 5% chance of coming through the next two years; with a transplant from Vicki he'd have a 40% chance, if it worked. He could of course end up further brain damaged, with tight skin, cataracts. Maybe we should take the chance because of *my* need of *him*. He asks if I have anyone to talk to; I say I'll go and see Duncan and he says he couldn't think of anyone better, he has a lot of experience in these situations.

Just a few words knock my whole world sideways. Maxine makes me coffee, helps me get myself together before I collect Adam and come home. I follow their advice and have a stiff drink. How can one ignore the leukaemia . . .

Phone George and say, I need you. He comes, and when he asks why, I tell him and he says, Oh Dr Evelyn told me all that on the phone, what's your problem? We're seeing Dr Evelyn and maybe the man who does the adult transplants at the JR, on Saturday 31st, the day he's taking Adam on the boat again.

Talk to Briony through a hole in the fence when I walk Sheba, tell her everything, and that I hope to see Duncan and am seeing Nick to talk about it. Duncan phones back and asks if I can go over tomorrow – say, Yes please, I need you after today's little session.

Wednesday 21 March

Mr Dinton works with Adam for about two hours – I'm surprised he could take so much. We go to Gerrards Cross, leave Adam happily with Thea while I go on to Duncan's.

He is so kind. He tries to explain to me that there are times when, if you love someone, you have to accept that maybe three months of being secure and happy in a loving environment is a better thing for them than say 30 years of life which is uncertain, full of frustration, unpleasant treatment and unhappiness. Leukaemia is an unpleasant disease, the treatment is unpleasant – what is the purpose of dragging Adam through this for an uncertain future? He of course knows as well as anyone Adam's odd medical history prior to the leukaemia, knows the uncertainty of his future life anyway. I feel I can put Adam through chemotherapy; I am almost certain I couldn't put him through the terrors and isolation of transplantation, but I can't look on that as deciding I want him to die. I'm in an absolute turmoil and, selfishly, I can't imagine my life without Adam, although of course the decision has to be made for his benefit, not because I have a need of him.

Monday 26 March
The last few days have been almost unbearable. I went to see the Vicar: the medical profession can achieve some terrible things; morally, when should one let them do what they can, and when should one draw the line? He also is extremely kind. He knew Adam almost died when he was six, and how worried I've been for Adam's adult life. I've discussed with him my rather wild ideas about trying to initiate some sort of smallholding scheme which would give Adam and others like him sheltered living as well as the dignity of work, among the soothing and spiritually-healing contact with animals and plants. He knows how I worried that after my death Adam might, through no fault of his own but simply as a misfit in our society, spend parts of his life either in prison or in psychiatric wards, simply because people are frightened of those who see things, understand things, in a different way, and their only answer is to remove such people from their day-to-day consciousness. How hurt and bewildered Adam would be, how vulnerable. When people enjoy a cute child and say in their delight, What a shame he has to grow up, they don't know what they are saying – some, like Peter Pan, don't.

The Vicar, knowing something of the background, says, Why on earth consider dragging Adam back yet again; surely this time 'the loving thing to do' (Duncan's phrase) would be to let Adam go. Duncan led me by the nose to that point, didn't actually say it, but it's obviously what he thinks, too. The hospital chaplain was no help: he said, Decide ignoring the brain damage. Really, I feel one can't ignore anything; one has to look at the situation as a whole or how can one possibly hope to arrive at a considered judgement. Nick was kind but George did most of the talking. I took George back to see the Vicar too. The dreadful thing is that this terrible decision has to be made by us and we are so emotionally involved we're the least likely to make a logical decision.

Justin has been here since Friday, seems much more relaxed and smiles at me.

George takes me out to dinner on Saturday so we can talk away from the young, and we have this incredible conversation about whether Adam should live or die. Across a table for two, candles, flowers, George says he could not make a decision which would result in death. I am thinking that a short life is not necessarily an incomplete one. We all want for our children a life of happiness, surrounded by people who love them, an easy death when the time comes. We have the opportunity to guarantee this for Adam and in a way it's beautiful: poor Vicki will have to take the big gamble, like George and me. George says if that's the way I feel, why don't I want to have numberless children and shoot them all before they reach the age of ten or thereabouts. Stupid. I don't feel I could make a decision which might result in Adam's surviving, further damaged. I don't want to cling on to Adam for selfish reasons, and I couldn't bear to see him suffer and know I was responsible for it – is that selfish too? Adam seems to think he will die soon and isn't afraid, so why should I be? I'm frightened of pain – physical and mental; George is frightened of death. I'm not, because I do believe in life going on after this world.

I remember the donkeys. When we adopted Fred Donkey, we knew he was very old. Then we felt sorry for him, alone in our paddock, so when someone asked if we would take on another donkey we welcomed Bill as a friend for Fred. Two years or so later, George and I had been out during the morning, leaving the children with the au pair at home. On our return Vicki, who was then nine, rushed up to us in floods of tears – poor Fred had died, poor Fred, she was so sorry for Fred. Adam, then six, who had been the one to discover and diagnose this condition in a calm and matter of fact manner, was furious at his sister's reaction. He said, Fred's all right, he's dead, don't cry for him. It's poor Bill, who has no friend now. Bill was indeed distraught, and I was full of admiration for this so-called mentally-handicapped child who had cut through the obvious reaction to one which, once he had pointed it out, was even more obvious.

Dr Morrison says we don't have to make a decision yet, we could continue chemotherapy, let him go through relapse into second remission and then decide. I don't believe this: they said originally that a second remission was extremely unlikely. Obviously a transplant would stand a better chance of success if performed while he were as fit as possible. I think this is a gentle way of approaching George, and I appreciate it. He says if we do have a transplant done, they'd do it here for him, on 4B, it'd be so much nicer for him to know the nurses. He's such a compassionate man – the children usually go to the Westminster for transplants. He apologises for Dr Evelyn's little speech, tells me how upset Maxine was. George thinks I just over-reacted; after all, he told him the same thing over the phone and he managed not to let it interfere with his routine.

He certainly concentrated our minds, which is no doubt what he intended.

Dr Morrison thinks Adam will have between twelve and eighteen months of enjoyable life on chemotherapy.

I ask George for more of his time for Adam. Must also ask him for something expensive for him, something which it would please him to give his son. He's always said he lives at such a pace, works so hard, for Adam, so he'll have tremendous adjustments to make, afterwards.

Victoria and Justin disappear off into student lodgings in Oxford.

13

Tuesday 27 March
Today started badly with Adam announcing he was *not* going into the Clinic, they'd only want to take his blood again and without his blood he'd die. Spend a long time explaining gently for the millionth time why this is not so, and that blood samples are necessary. We get there in the end, Dr Keith takes blood sample and gives vincristine – it doesn't cost him anything for dud attempts today. Prednisone for five days, no other treatment because his blood count is still low.

Joanne gives us some sponsorship forms – her husband is running in the London Marathon – Adam and I take them around the village later and get a good response. The fire escape entrance to the hospital is open again – a large greenhouse structure has been erected around the fire escape, which Dr Morrison told us cost £50,000. No wonder haematology needs to raise funds from things like this to acquire their £5,000 blood-typing machine.

Wednesday 28 March
Adam seems tired again. After lunch we visit a farm at Grendon Underwood – Stuart is a schoolfriend of Adam's. It's a proper old-fashioned farm (I mean that in the nicest possible way!) with a full dairy herd, an impressive bull, new calves; sheep and new-born lambs – the very new ones are all knubbly, only the slightly older ones are soft and woolly. There are pigs and piglets in all sizes, and a massive boar. It's a delightful place and they are lovely people too, give us tea and say we can come again.

Thursday 29 March
Adam cycles down to the Church with me to tidy Granny's grave, so he has a little fresh air and exercise, but mostly we read, play shut-the-box which is an arithmetic game. We both feel a little dozy – maybe because we have the gas heater on.

Friday 30 March
Adam seems really bright and has a good session with Mr Dinton. They study the world map, trying to trace the route George will embark upon next week. It's difficult for Adam to understand, on the flat! As George went westward last time, I think he should go the other way round this time, give himself an opportunity to unwind.

We later visit Grandad, who looks florid and puffs a lot. I have such dreadful resentful feelings about him: he sits there like a toad in his room, consuming emotion, complaining about the staff, the other residents and the food, yet he eats so much he's bursting out of his clothes. After a bout of these dreadful thoughts I'm filled with remorse and visit him again with sherry, biscuits, chocolate and cigarettes, listen to the same old stories, hold his hand and come home so sorry for him but feeling if he manages to outlive Adam I'll strangle him with my own hands. I'm terrible, wicked, I just can't work out these feelings.

George comes home and we spend this ludicrous evening with me trying to discuss life, death, transplants, and George on another tack altogether.

He's now in favour of a transplant, says he doesn't want to feel he is shedding his responsibilities. I'm against transplantation. I think that without it we have Adam for probably a year or two and we can make sure it's a happy time for him and that the end is gentle.

I dream of being drowned, being chased, finding someone has removed the entire contents of my house. Don't go much on Freud; too many snakes, not enough ladders.

Saturday 31 March
Freezing, snow on the Chilterns and a bitter wind, everything including me grey and miserable. Even cockerel hardly crows. Drop Adam off at the Burretts' then George and I go to the JR to see Dr Evelyn. He strikes just the right note and we all end up agreeing no transplantation, we'll keep Adam on the chemotherapy; he says he's sure we've made the right decision.

Bring Vicki and Justin home for the weekend with their laundry, get Adam and George ready for their boating trip – woolly hats, scarves, mitts, hot-water bottles, sleeping bags, chocolate biscuits for Sailor the dog, and Adam takes his fishing line to trail, he promised Mr Burrett a fish.

Spend the afternoon going round the village with sponsorship forms again – it takes a long time because so many people haul me in to talk. Get home with no feeling in toes, ears or fingers.

George had assured me that the boat is warm.

Sunday 1 April
Sunny but even colder. After communion the Vicar asks me if we've made a decision: tell him. Vicki and Justin make a roaring fire – it gets too hot for me in the sitting room. They leave before 6:00; George returns with Adam almost immediately. Adam couldn't fish, he tells me, because it's the closed season. Sailor fell in – luckily he's a good swimmer – and he showered everyone when he was heaved out again. They saw lots of ducks and swans but forgot to throw them the stale bread they took for the purpose – they carefully brought it back home again. They went out to dinner at a fancy waterside inn and Bill ate *snails*. Adam says he still feels strange, like yesterday, sort of dizzy.

Monday 2 April
Adam still feels strange so I put off Mr Dinton who was quite glad; he'd been on a golfing weekend and also felt strange. Adam cheers up enough to come play outside with Lennie for an hour or so later, and we discover Little Black Bantam is sitting on eggs.

Tuesday 3 April
Adam's blood count well up so he's back on half-strength chemotherapy and no Clinic next week. He's sorry about the tablets, glad not to have to go in next Tuesday.

Wednesday 4 April
Mr Dinton brings a globe which makes George's round-the-world route much more comprehensible, and spends more than an hour with Adam. Afterwards we visit Grandad, whose legs are bad again. The doctor says he's not to push Edith's wheelchair any more and he feels low.

Peter offers to cut the grass for me and trails Adam about

in the trailer behind the baby tractor for a couple of hours which they both enjoy immensely. Takes twice as long to cut the grass that way, but it's far more fun!

Thursday 5 April

Poor Sheba doesn't get enough attention. My laughing dog isn't laughing any more. She's unhappy. She isn't allowed upstairs, but has taken to following me everywhere, crying, trying to get my attention with her heavy expressive paw. She even came and whimpered next to the bath last night. She is badly in need of a good grooming, more walks. She's off her food, kicks her dish around, sleeps right behind my feet when I'm working in the kitchen – one day I'll step back, fall over her and break something important. She makes me feel so guilty – one assumes such a responsibility when one acquires an animal, they are so utterly dependent.

Off to leave Adam happily with Karen while I go and see Duncan. Feel I'm being an awful bore but he's wonderful, so easy to talk to, and asks me to go through the whole thing, who we've seen, how we feel, whether George and I agree, step by step. He envisages taking it one stage further: chemotherapy is unpleasant and if we've decided against a transplant for Adam why continue chemotherapy; perhaps opt out of the trials after a year when we'll have had an extra six months or so to give Adam a good time. Why prolong the agony? It makes sense but my emotions are way behind.

He tells me I should have a lover who would cuddle me and make it all seem bearable – a lovely prescription; unfortunately I can't think of an appropriate dispensing chemist!

Tells me to come and talk to him again soon.

Adam has unaccountably wet himself in Karen's car. She isn't flustered, lends Adam some of Brian's gardening trousers to come home in – and then I manage to come home without the bag of wet clothes. Most embarrassing, but Karen is super when I phone, just says, Well, we'll launder and post.

Friday 6 April

Visit Grandad after Adam's lessons. He's still confined to his room with a bad leg, and will let me know whether or not to collect him on Sunday. He's pleased with the things we took in for him. Old folk seem to smell of biscuits, like very small children smell of bread and butter. Adam says on our way home how sorry he is for Grandad, poor Grandad, he ought to be dead.

After lunch Adam walks Sheba, goes to help Chris with his horses and calves. Nick phones to ask how Adam is and whether we've come to any decision. Tell him Adam is very well at the moment and we've decided against a transplant. He says he feels George dominated the conversation when we met so maybe he related more to George than to me and would I like to talk to him again. Say I think the next stage is to see Dr Evelyn again, then I'd like to make an appointment with him.

Adam asks me a couple of times today if I'm sure I'm his mother. Say, Yes, darling, I was most certainly there when you were born, Daddy was too – why? But he'll only say, Oh, I just wondered. Aren't I behaving like his mother?

Monday 9 April

Uneventful, rather chilly weekend. Adam was extremely energetic helping in the garden, walking Sheba, out on his bike, helping Chris in the fields with his calves and horses. He finishes and posts his letters thanking Stuart's parents for their hospitality and telling Mrs Wolf and the class about his visit to Stuart's farm. He thinks Stuart is very lucky to live on a farm.

The nursing home phoned to say Grandad had a funny turn and is on bed rest, can't come over on Sunday, but I'm not to worry. Vicki and Justin in Oxford, so Adam and I have roast duck to ourselves.

When Adam seems well and it's daylight I'm all right. After dark the snakes in my stomach come back and the whole mess swirls round inside my head and I'm frightened, so frightened of the entire unspeakable situation. I feel so isolated and out of my depth. How on earth am I to find the strength to help Adam – and George – be happy and enjoy whatever life we have left together?

After Adam's lessons today we go and see Grandad, take him some cold roast duck and a large bar of chocolate. It's quite a shock to see him: dishevelled, disorientated and very confused. He recognised Adam but thought he was alone at first, didn't seem to see me. He clambers in and out of bed, shows me his leg four or five times – the swelling seems to have gone down. He swears he's had nothing to eat and no one's been near him for days. I couldn't understand half he said.

Send Adam back to wait in the car while I go talk to Matron. He hasn't had another stroke as I had thought, but they think it was a transient ischaemic attack which is a pre-stroke thing and a stroke may follow, the next few days will tell.

I ask their attitude on fighting for survival – whether they preserve a flicker of life at all costs or whether they accept that there comes a time when this is wrong and someone ought to be allowed to go gently, with dignity, because their natural time has come. Oh yes, she says, if it comes to the point where a decision must be taken Doctor discusses the situation with the next-of-kin and states quite clearly that she thinks no further active treatment is indicated. But that it very rarely comes to that stage, and Grandad could recover or just as easily have a major stroke and die very quickly; they'll do all they can to keep him comfortable.

Tuesday 10 April
No Clinic! Adam and I take Mr Burrett to the Cottage Hospital for his therapy, Mrs Burrett to shop.

Phone to ask after Grandad and speak to the doctor, who says it is definitely a transient ischaemic attack and there's nothing but good nursing care and wait-and-see; no need to send for George, he could get better but equally could go in the next ten minutes. Poor Grandad, I do hope he's feeling peaceful. I feel so guilty for all the nasty resentful thoughts I've had about him.

I make an appointment to take Sheba to the vet. tomorrow. Poor Sheba, I can't neglect her any more but I simply don't have the time or the energy to spend three hours twice a week grooming her. She won't go for walks with anyone other than Adam or me, and she doesn't even get the company she needs either. She's so much my dog I'm sure she'd never fit in with another family at her age. I know something has to give, and it simply can't be me. This is the logical decision, she's certainly not happy and things are likely to get worse around here rather than better. I feel absolutely rotten, a Judas betraying those big trusting brown eyes. I cry and she licks me with sympathy which makes it worse.

Adam spends more time out than in today, comes back healthily tired after helping Chris in the fields; hearty supper, bath and bed.

Wednesday 11 April

Didn't sleep much, thinking about today. Get up early and take Sheba for a long walk through the fields with tears streaming down my face. Give her a good breakfast. Adam waits in the car while I take Sheba in to the vet., have hysterics and make a real exhibition of myself while paying him £15 to kill my dog. Adam knew Sheba wasn't happy. I tell him the vet. found a tumour and this was the kindest thing to do; we cry together. My duplicity makes it so much worse for me.

We go to visit Grandad who is even more disorientated and feeling dreadful. Tells me he had a visit from Adam and Adam this morning but he hasn't seen Adam since – we haven't a clue what he's talking about. He wants to come home, holds my hands and begs me to bring him home, he'll feel better at home. How's Adam, he hasn't seen Adam for so long. Stroke his hand and tell him he has to get stronger before he can come home. It's terrible and neither Adam nor I can take too much.

Adam waits in the car while Matron suggests it may be the result of a secondary tumour on the brain but there's no point in distressing him with further investigations as there's nothing to be done anyway other than keep him comfortable. He pushed his commode into the bathroom last night, locked the door and then fell – they had quite a bit of sorting out to do. He trampled the cold duck and chocolate we took him into the carpet – he's so restless his room is in chaos 20 minutes after being cleaned, he takes the mattress off the bed and everything. His teeth have been found, but they, his watch and specs. are in constant peril. I'm not to bring Adam with me any more, it's not right that he should see his grandfather in such a state. I feel sick.

Pauline comes to lunch; steak and salad and Adam eats well. George phones from Hong Kong. Tell him about his father and Sheba – that Sheba had a tumour – he's very upset and tells me I'm doing well. I don't feel I am. He says he can't do anything about his father's condition so he doesn't think he'll break off his business trip and come home, especially as the doctor said it wasn't necessary. I'm disappointed but his attitude is logical and that's George.

Late this evening the nursing home phones to say Grandad fell and cut his head on a radiator. I don't need to come in tonight but I did know he was very restless, didn't I?

Adam decides he wants another dog, *now*; spits and swears about it. Tell him we can't have another dog till after the summer as we want to be free to go away on holiday and on day trips and it wouldn't be fair. He calms down, he respects the needs of animals.

Oh glory, what a day.

Thursday 12 April

Phone the nursing home first thing to see how Grandad is. He spent a peaceful night but I did realise what sort of state he was in during the evening, didn't I? He smeared his faeces all over himself, the carpet, television, inside drawers, down walls – everything was scrubbed down with a very strong disinfectant but she must apologise for having to take the carpet up. Feel sick again, clammy with cold perspiration.

See Chris and Willow, ask if there's anything Adam could help them with while I nip up to see Grandad before George phones. Yes, he can help them with the horses. Willow says I should tell George to come home, this is all too much and it's *his* father, but I can't.

Mr Burrett appears and says Adam has told him the sad news; I ask Grandad or Sheba and he says, My God, and starts crying, most upset for us, muttering about people who help people getting it all and rotten people getting away with it. Offers to have Adam for me, and whatever other help he or Mrs Burrett can give. They are lovely people. I make my escape into the car, shaking because I dread seeing Grandad, and I don't feel nearly as good as Mr Burrett obviously thinks I am.

Grandad cleaned up, in bed and fairly docile; grabs my hand, cries and talks nonsense. The word 'music' seems to be used on the many instances he loses a word. He doesn't know where he is, how long he's been there, or what happened. It bothers him, but not as much as the music which he can't hear. He says Mother hasn't been in much – I'm interested she's been in at all, as she died a year ago. Strokes my hand and wants me to bring him home. I see 'home' as a synonym for 'peace' and hope I can.

Get home in time to finish fixing lunch for Ben and Jane – I'd made pancakes last night, shoved a chicken casserole and potato-pud into the oven before going out. They add an element of reality to the day and Adam eats well as he tends to do in company. He shows them the ducks so he's nicely out of the way when George phones and I have to tell him his father is occasionally demented but no further advance on the medical prognosis or advice. He's just going out to dinner, he's in a hurry, so he'll think about it and call me back.

He does so at 6:15 – 1.15 a.m. in Hong Kong. After a lot of transcontinental heavy breathing at £5 a minute or whatever it is, he decides to continue his business trip as there's nothing he can do here, after all. True; I can't argue. Irrationally, I'm disappointed he doesn't want to be here and at least try to support *me*, even if he can't do anything practical for anyone else. Does he feel I don't need support? Does he want me to say, you must come home, we need you? Why don't I know this man I married? I try to feel I'm supporting him by not screaming for help as soon as there's a crisis, glad he has the confidence that I can give him the facts and cope by myself.

At least Adam is happy today – he enjoyed spending so much time helping Chris and Willow with their animals.

I think I'm getting a lesson from the Almighty, direct, with graphic illustrations: there are worse things in life than death.

14

Friday 13 April
Can't seem to keep myself clean enough no matter how often I bath, change clothes, bed linen. I expect it's the result of stress – Pauline advised some vitamin tablets called Ladycare. I'd love to be able to think vitamin tablets could fix everything for me! She also thinks I could manage better without George round my neck demanding attention all the time.

Adam and I finish his jigsaw before his teacher comes. He has a happy day – it's sunny and we are too, somehow. After lunch he rides in the trailer as Peter cuts the grass for me.

Grandad slightly more coherent. Strokes my hand all the time, cries and says he and Mother were always friends and what it's going to be like after this he doesn't know. Tells me one minute George has been such a help this week, and the next that he doesn't know why George hasn't been in. Explain several times that George is away, first Hong Kong now Australia; he can't grasp it. Wants to know how I manage the rabbits, how will they carry on with him laid up. What rabbits? He wants a cigarette so I light him one. He seems to have no spatial concept, can barely hold it, tries to put it into his mouth the wrong way round and then into his ear. I hold it for him to puff a few times, then say we'd better put it out or he'll burn himself. Oh yes, Katherine, thank you, Katherine, so humbly. He cries again when I tell him I think he's better than yesterday. Stay three-quarters of an hour and hate myself for not spending longer with him, but I just can't take too much.

Adam puts the chicks and ducks to bed for me – I'm so pleased he can manage, and that he thought of it – he knows what difficulty I had with them yesterday. He wet his pants in the orchard; wonder if he has a little infection.

I come to the conclusion that George doesn't like me because I make myself do things he can't do and so make him feel subconsciously guilty and ashamed. Maybe Freud has something after all: life does have too many snakes and not enough ladders.

Saturday 14 April
Another beautiful sunny day, and Adam lounges round in pyjamas, distinctly off. I can't leave him on his own like this, Chris and Willow are busy, so I ring the nursing home. Grandad much the same, says Sister, they feed and toilet him and manage pretty much to keep him clean; he's still going in and out of these attacks. Explain I won't be able to visit today; she says they understand my position, give it a miss and don't feel guilty. I know he doesn't remember from one moment to the next so why do I feel so bad about not going to hold his hand for a few minutes?

Adam and I do puzzles, cut-outs and watch television together. He doesn't know how or why he doesn't feel well, but hardly moves from the sofa all day. Hardly eats, either. Cat seems to understand, curls up beside him and purrs beautifully when he strokes her, 'starting up her purr motor'.

Sunday 15 April
Adam feels poorly, very demanding this morning. We do more puzzles. He spends the afternoon watching television alone – swears at me, is generally nasty if I go near him. Won't let me go see Grandad even though he doesn't want me himself, *hates* Grandad, and me, and doctors and nurses . . . I catch up on a few boring jobs around the house.

George phones from Melbourne to see if everything's all right! Can't explain Adam's behaviour to him, simply say he isn't feeling well and is being difficult.

Monday 16 April
Adam brighter – goes to let out the chicks and ducks while I cook his breakfast sausages. Lennie appears and they go off to play together so I go and see Grandad, taking some daffodils from the garden and some chocolate. He tries to squirrel them away under the bedclothes; fish them out a couple of times, but have the nasty feeling they'll find chocolate-coated daffodils in his bed next time they change him. Less spatial concept – he reaches for my hand and misses by a good six inches. Seems less able to see and hear well. Knows my name but appears

not to know who I am, where I fit into the scheme of things. Says he hasn't seen anything of George or his young lady. Has George been busy with his music?

Adam comes home demanding a picnic to take off across the fields with Lennie. George phones to ask if everything's all right. Say no, it isn't.

Nick calls while Adam's helping Chris with the calves, talks to me about transient ischaemic attacks (and spells them for me) but can't add much to what has already been said. He confirms my sweaty shaky turns are probably due to stress but doesn't have any suggestions as to how I can get myself together and cope better. He's coming to lunch again next week – bearing in mind last time, I have every admiration for him and am so grateful. Adam still has nightmares about doctors and the more he sees of them in congenial surroundings as nice guys the better, in addition to the fact that he eats better when the company adds up to more than me.

Tuesday 17 April

Adam keen to go to Clinic, says he wants to see that smiley baby again – Michael's baby sister.

While Adam's with Maxine, I tell Dr Evelyn he seemed so much better when he was off chemotherapy for three weeks; that he obviously doesn't have much faith in the efficacy of the drugs with such a low prognosis, so was there much point in continuing chemotherapy? He says, Good question. First, he may have felt better then because he took a long time to recover from the effects of radiotherapy and is now in the second six-month phase of his treatment, not simply because he was off treatment for three weeks. Secondly, he would like to continue to treat him because he *may* be one of the very few who come through, and although he knows I worry about Adam's life when I'm no longer around to look after him, I could well live to be 80 and therefore able to care for him for 35 more years. Have I discussed this with George and does he have another woman? I say no. He says we can wait for Adam to relapse before deciding whether or not to continue treatment. I feel that is simply procrastination; the point is, I want him to have a *good* life, no matter how long it is. He says if we stopped chemotherapy he'd relapse within six months but he may well anyway, and that if we decide to withdraw Adam from the trials they'd respect our wishes.

Adam disappears into the fields with Chris again for the afternoon. Knowing Chris must be the next best thing to living on a farm.

Wednesday 18 April
Find Grandad in the psychiatrics' sitting room and he almost falls out of his chair in his effort to greet me, grasps my hands and massages half-masticated biscuit into them, calls me Vicki. Has his coffee in a baby's feeding cup. He has a very sore eye into which Sister has just put some ointment. He keeps rubbing it and hopes George will come soon and help him take the cucumber out of his eye. He doesn't seem to know who his feet belong to.

Come across Matron on my way out. She says I do understand he needs the supervision possible only in that sitting room, don't I, and that he poured water into all his drawers while looking for his goldfish. (His goldfish expired some time ago, probably from over-feeding, although he suspected sabotage.) His sore eye may mean a secondary cancer in the brain – pressure. There's a drug which could temporarily alleviate the pressure if that is it and which won't harm him if it isn't. He has so little co-ordination I'm surprised he can home in on his eye often enough to rub it sore. I do hope he doesn't go on too long in this distressing state, poor old man.

George phones, seems shocked his father has to use that sitting room; I thought I'd said enough for him to understand.

Maxine comes over and I talk to her a lot. She thinks I should get away for a few days without Adam, talks of Helen House, offers to come 'babysit' if I'd like to go out one evening. She's so kind, but there's really nowhere I want to go.

Thursday 19 April
Dental check-up. Dentist looks at Adam's yellow teeth and asks if he's on a wide-spectrum antibiotic. He is; so that is what has discoloured his teeth. He brushes it off, tells Adam he has very good teeth. Thank God. I have to go back for a filling. Of course.

We both rest for a while after lunch. We see the first swallows sitting on the telegraph wires. Adam helps Chris again, is so bright and cheerful he's an absolute joy.

Good Friday 20 April
Don't wake early enough to go to Church, having spent a good deal of the night feeling lost, lonely. Adam wakes tired and we spend the day playing and doing puzzles.

Thea phones and says she'll pray for us. Pauline phones to ask if we'd like to run down to Milford for the day, but over bank holidays I'd sooner stay close to home than commit myself to long-haul drives, especially with an unwell child.

Just before 5:00 Adam livens up, gets dressed and goes off dog-walking with Chris, so I shoot off to see Grandad. He tells me he's all ready, when can we go home, he's longing to go home, tears and Oh it's so painful. His eye looks better but he has a shrunken look; it's not so long since I had to buy him larger shirts because he was bursting out of his clothes, now he has the appearance of a tortoise stretching neck and head out of an uncomfortable carapace.

I associate his use of the word 'home' more and more with 'peace', 'death'.

A girl comes in to feed him his supper, tells me he had a full three-course lunch too, there's nothing wrong with his appetite.

I wish I could disassociate myself like George can; life must be so much easier if you can pay a few bills, make some phone calls and feel satisfied that you've done your duty. Why do I have to have a conscience? They're such uncomfortable things to have around!

Help Adam have his third shave after his bath.

Saturday 21 April
When Vicki rings I tell her about Grandad and Sheba; she's very upset and says she and Justin will be back tonight till Monday.

It's a beautiful day. Adam helps me do some gardening and we hear the cuckoo for the first time. It's the sort of day to go picking dandelions for wine-making, but the needs of the garden are more pressing. I've seen people picking dandelion flowers on the roadside verges, but I prefer to pick mine in the fields; the Charolais, in my opinion, add a little je ne sais quoi which is vastly superior to carbon monoxide as an additive. Dandelion-gathering is not an occupation Adam finds particularly entertaining, so I'll skip it, this year.

Although I never buy cabbage plants, they keep appearing in the garden. My family won't eat broad beans and I think Mr Burrett feels a period of deprivation, in spite of the purple sprouting broccoli we all love. Anyway, I have such ambivalent feelings concerning these flourishing cabbages: I don't even like cutting them – so many things live inside them it's like destroying a whole universe – and I can't possibly bring myself to serve the remains of Home to so many creatures. George once reprimanded me, said I was losing my sense of adventure. The fact remains, cabbage is one of the few things I would rather buy than grow, but equally I don't want to upset dear Mr Burrett, so I find myself cutting cabbages, looking over my shoulder, and shoving the wretched things into the dustbin!

Vicki and Justin back for supper – pork chops and celebration wine. She's learned a lot, living in digs, and I think she should do so for longer before taking herself off to the other side of the world. It sounds so far away, and so lonely, Australia.

They suggest they all come to Church with me in the morning – I'm so pleased.

Easter Sunday 22 April

Beautiful to have the three of them beside me in Church this morning. After, we drop Justin and Adam at home while I take Vicki to see her Grandad, which she finds quite difficult. The ladies take him to the loo, undo him, leave him for a while then call, Have you finished, Mr Adair? He says, I don't know, come and try and see what you think. The ladies laugh, say, Better than the telly, a laugh a minute – they're so natural, unembarrassed, loving even, I feel it gives *me* strength to know there are such good, caring people in the world. Poor Vicki laughs almost hysterically, this is upsetting for her. He has definitely shrunk; he has his teeth in today, and they don't fit any more, either. How does it happen?

Vicki and Justin keep the washing-machine going all day, and inspire Adam who is more lively, outgoing. They all eat with relish everything I put in front of them, and then refills. I enjoy them all tremendously. A very good day.

Easter Monday 23 April

Adam, feeling really friendly and chatty, appears in my room fully-dressed well before 6:00 this morning. He understands that waking up is a lengthy process for me, makes me coffee to assist the proceedings.

While Vicki and Justin are amusing Adam, I go to see Grandad. I deliberately go at different times, irregular days, so they can't keep track of me but I get a good idea of how they cope with Grandad and would know if he were in any way neglected. I have a nasty suspicious nature; it's quite uncalled-for, I couldn't fault them.

He's weak and wobbly after the strain of a bath, but knows me, says he wants to give me a present for all I've done for him; would I like some money from the moon! What a beautiful idea! He wants me to bring him some thorns to scratch a map with, and two more watches. I can't translate this at all. His room is in a state again which is not nice for him because in between these bouts of mania or whatever you call them he is reasonably with-it and realises he turned everything upside down. He still wants to know if I manage all right, will I bring him home now, how am I for money? I wonder who he thinks I am.

We drop Vicki and Justin off for their bus, then Adam and I have a picnic lunch in the garden. We amuse ourselves watching ants industriously rushing about between the blades of grass, carrying things around, passing messages to each other in code by tapping heads with their antennae. They have compound eyes but do not appear able to see, as they bumble around.

We lie on the picnic rug watching birds. Starlings are such vocal extroverts, seem to live life with such passion and careless enjoyment, they seem to be the Italians in our little Europe. The stout and serious blackbirds and thrushes, earnestly shopping around for the choicest food, I imagine as being black-skirted, head-scarved French and Belgian housewives; robins, the neat, orderly Swiss. Swallows aren't people though: trim, fast, streaking overhead in formation, they have to be fighter jets, just as the collared doves resemble the heavy, ungainly Lancaster bombers.

We steal a bantam egg to hold to our ears and hear the tap, tap, tapping and cheeping of the baby chick – very exciting!

It's a beautiful afternoon, we share so much from so little – it could so easily have gone unnoticed.

Tuesday 24 April

Before Clinic we do chicks and ducks and Adam discovers that Little Black Bantam has four or five babies hiding in her feathers, and more to come – he's egg-static!

Clinic takes ages – it's vincristine day so we have to wait for Dr Keith to come down from the Ward rather than go up to Joanne for the blood sample. Results take so long we end up going to 4B around 12:00 to wait. Maxine says Dr Evelyn blew a gasket and said Clinic Must Be Re-Organised. Blood count fine, continue ¾ treatment.

Rush to the chick house on our return, discover *nine* babies under Little Black Bantam! When Vicki returns we move the chick house onto fresh grass, put in fresh nestbox full of straw, put out finely-chopped hard-boiled egg – even if it does seem vaguely cannibalistic, chick crumbs, water. Vicki is also enthralled, she didn't see the last ones when they were babies, a teaspoonful of fluff and bounce, quite independent and capable of coping with life. Adam takes one carefully into the lane to show Chris and Willow, Briony and Ted, and anyone else he can find. Vicki goes to ask Mr Herbert if the cockerel will hurt the babies – is it all right to shut them all up together at night; he says it's okay. Pure joy.

Wednesday 25 April

Woken early by a furious swearing spitting Adam throwing the doorstop at my head, steaming, stamping, utterly *mad* because he can't find his sunglasses. Takes almost an hour to find them and calm him down.

We shop, and bump into his teacher, Mrs Wolf, which pleases Adam. Go on to see Grandad; Adam stays by the car talking to a little dog while I slip in. He seems so much saner now, I think the tablets are helping, therefore it must be a secondary tumour in the brain, they wouldn't make any difference if it wasn't. He feels in his pockets and says he hasn't any bicycles – I translate this and go fetch him a clean handkerchief from his room. He wants to know if the servants are helping me because they aren't doing much for him. Difficult, that.

Adam and I unshop, have toasted cheese sandwiches and salad outside for lunch while we watch the baby chicks – a delight, an illustration of the vigour of life. Adam keeps saying how he misses his Dad, when is his Dad coming back. Does he just want to share the miracle of the chicks, I wonder, or is he expecting something, and if so, what? I hope he won't be disappointed.

Thursday 26 April
Mother Bantam has hatched six babies, so it's fifteen altogether. Adam delighted, plans a series of further chick houses while I start dropping hints about Good Homes with Other People . . .

Nick comes to lunch and we eat outside in the sunshine with the corner of the tablecloth in the gravy. I do steak in wine and mushroom sauce, sautéed new potatoes, spinach salad with chicory and red peppers, croutons and bits of crispy bacon; creamy yoghurty thing for pudding. He admires chicks with gratifying enthusiasm (particularly when you remember his people are farmers) and is satisfyingly appreciative of lunch, which even I have to admit is ten times better than the last time he came. George phones; he'll be back Saturday. Nick says if we want to go and see him please do, and keep in touch anyway. He asks after Grandad and says it is quite likely that melanoma on the foot has turned itself into a secondary carcinoma of the brain.

He knows we've decided against transplantation for Adam and asks about my latest conversation with Dr Evelyn. Explain I told him Adam was so much better without the medication; that he doesn't seem to have much faith in chemotherapy, giving him only a 5% chance of living while on drugs, therefore what would he think about stopping chemotherapy, would the difference to the quality of life make it worthwhile? That he said he wanted to continue to treat Adam although he'd abide by our wishes, as he may be among the few to be cured. But, as Duncan said, they've done two-year trials and three-year trials, no one's done a six-month trial or a twelve-month one, he may be cured now. Without chemotherapy he'd relapse in six months but he may anyway, so why not let him feel as well as he can meanwhile if his time might be limited. Nick seems to understand the way I feel, even if he, like everyone else, has no answer. There are some questions which simply don't have an answer; you just have to do your best. Such a strong feeling of, is empathy the right word, emanates from that man. It makes me feel good, just knowing he's there.

Friday 27 April

Not much sleep last night. Vicki detected a spider in her room around midnight, and in lieu of much activity from me on hearing the news she woke Adam, who joined enthusiastically in a noisy, lengthy and ultimately unsuccessful spider hunt in her room. She kept her light on all night. I slept for a while after the seek-and-destroy exercise, woke again early.

Adam disappears on his bike, so I do chores and some shopping, see Grandad at tea time. He's tearful again, begging me to bring him home. Says he has nothing left to live for. Keeps on about food, or lack of same. More distressed than he has been for a week, and I don't know what to do about it.

Saturday 28 April

George arrives around midday with a big pile of laundry, two new computer games, perfume for Vicki and me, a hat and a gorilla mask for Adam.

Lunch in the garden, then we go and see Grandad (Adam stays in the car playing tapes). He rambles, dribbles, but knows us and transfers biscuits from my hand into his mouth perfectly although he makes a mess eating them. Reads the time as 8:00 instead of 4:00. Carries on at great length about music. George found it all a shock although I'd tried to prepare him.

Supper all together, the four of us: lovely.

Sunday 29 April

Don't sleep till dawn and when I do I have nightmares about losing Adam. A policeman calls to tell me he's lost, some place 30 miles away. He drives me there and I rush about searching. It's night-time and I'm in and out of brilliant light from arc-lamps and absolute dark – getting desperate. It's a vast building site in a huge area with big machines I don't understand, holes and mountains of earth, I'm stumbling around looking for him. Why can't I find him, I love him so much I should *know* where he is. I didn't know Adam was lost till Authority told me so.

Sunny but cold. I started to plough through George's mass of laundry, help Adam write his diary, watch birds.

Adam listens to Jimmy Saville on the radio while he helps me to prepare lunch – he likes chopping up carrots and courgettes – and every record Jimmy Saville plays is one Adam has in his room. We start laughing about it, and I tease him, Come now, Adam, even if this Jimmy Saville fellow is a friend of yours, you should *ask* me before inviting him to do his radio programme from your room using your records. He giggles and denies it, but each succeeding record is one he has in his collection. I ask how many people he has squirrelled away upstairs, and what will they want for lunch? He can hardly answer through his laughter; yet another record from his collection comes on the air, until we are both helpless with laughter and tears.

George goes to see his father; Vicki comes down just before lunch which George insists we eat outside. George oils the baby tractor for me, Peter later cuts the grass; I feel cared for, for a moment. I iron, iron, iron; I'm tired. George asks what I plan to do next weekend, bank holiday. Say, Nothing in particular, what are you and Vicki doing? I didn't mean to in the least, but I started a full-blown row with that; they both get abusive, particularly George, who storms out, leaving me in floods of tears, all over nothing.

15

Monday 30 April
A bad night and today doesn't seem at first to have a lot going for it, but then Mr Dinton says Adam worked well and agrees he'd now benefit from a return to school. Ring Education Department and school, fix for Adam to go back next week; I'll take him and fetch him home at lunch time to begin with, we'll see how he goes. He's very pleased.

George phones to suggest taking Adam on the boat for a long weekend 11 May, then spends ages telling me how difficult it would be.

Visit Grandad, wheel him into the garden. Surprise, surprise, he wants me to take him home. When I say he'll have to get stronger before I can do that, he says, Well, you can stay with me then – so he is getting a trifle more logical!

Mr Burrett drops hints about not being able to carry on in the garden much longer. Arthritis. I wonder if I'll have to move; it's all becoming a bit much.

Adam and I walk in the fields. He laughs at me, stumbling on the rough ground and trying to dodge the thistles – I've got sandals on and it isn't comfortable. He holds my hand and tries to guide me between them. We swing along, happy in the early evening sun, but there is still the shadow of the dog . . .

There are some new bullocks in the next field, young ones with broad black and white panda faces, soft brown eyes full of curiosity; they bounce up to look at us, and line up three or four deep rather like an audience, gazing up at us with expectancy, so I start a song and dance routine. Adam sees the situation exactly, laughs and loves it – until he notices a couple of figures at the far end of the field also watching me with curiosity. I don't mind being caught entertaining the bullocks – and they are entertained, vastly – but Adam becomes embarrassed at his idiotic mother, I'm to behave myself. I stand rebuked, and we amble back in a more sedate manner, both of us appreciating the restorative qualities of the countryside, pleasantly tired.

Tuesday 1 May
To Clinic early. Adam is so good now about having his blood sample taken; he hangs onto my hand, leans against me and takes a deep breath while I stroke his face and talk to him. Joanne has a lovely easy manner with the children and chatters away about her animals while she does it, quickly.

Dr Morrison says Adam is doing well, up to full treatment, come back in two weeks. Maxine sends Adam off to pharmacy while she tells me Joe died on Friday, a little more than two weeks after his transplant. At home, Adam goes off on his bike; I spend two hours praying and trying to compose a letter to Joe's parents.

Wednesday 2 May
Ted and Briony come to supper and we have a lovely time – they're uplifting people. Adam eats well.

Thursday 3 May
Play with Adam then he stays here and colours a doodleart meticulously while I go to the dentist and zip in for a quick visit with Grandad. His co-ordination seems a lot better, his mind much worse. You understand the words but not what he means. His clarinet hasn't arrived, he was glad to take Adam in a taxi last night but doesn't think he will tonight; he's going skating, and oh the pain, he's miserable, so miserable. I'm assured he has maximum analgesics but I know also that state of mind can induce pain, real pain. What I can do for him I just don't know, and leave when I start feeling so knotted inside I feel sick, which is my usual way of timing visits. He's usually had enough by then, too.

Friday 4 May
Adam feeling sleepy and floppy so ring Mr Dinton and suggest he wouldn't do much work in the circumstances, perhaps best not to come. He agrees and we part with expressions of mutual esteem and goodwill.

Shop, unshop, have lunch. I cut the grass while Adam rests in front of the television. George rings to say he'll be down tomorrow – everything's so normal I could scream because it isn't!

Saturday 5 May
George arrives for lunch and is in a reasonably cheerful mood. In the afternoon he and Adam sleep; I garden. Wouldn't it be nice if they could bottle the scent of newly-cut grass?

We all go out for dinner. Vicki seems a trifle tense, suddenly starts crying and says she has a pain in her left breast which shoots up into her head. George keeps clutching his middle and assuming an expression of agony with appropriate sound-effects. However, Adam and I enjoy our dinner. They have a special sea-food dinner next Friday; George books a table for us.

Sunday 6 May
George takes his father for a drive, says he's lucid but heavily sedated, which is certainly not the way I saw him last. Hope he's more peaceful.

Over lunch Vicki starts making remarks I can only consider calculated to be provocative, and riles her father. Corner him in the kitchen, say I know she's not thinking straight, please help her to be constructive, give her a few pointers instead of ridiculing her. He gets her to work on some costings and making notes about various things concerning her proposed trip to Australia.

Monday 7 May
George has groaned and puffed a lot this weekend. He says he's swollen around his middle, back and front, that there's something seriously wrong with him; he's seen a doctor who said, Hmmm there's a lot of it about, don't worry it may go away. I don't believe it! Anyway, he's been touchy, bad tempered, wanting sympathy and lots of sleep. I try, but my supply of sympathy is running rather low. He goes off to a meeting after lunch.

Wednesday 9 May
Adam goes back to school. I drive him in and collect him at 12:15, take Vicki to the doctor's and visit Grandad in between. I know it's extremely unlikely that there's anything seriously

wrong with her breast, but I've learned that the terrible things which only happen to other people can happen to us, haven't I. She's okay, Briony is reassuring.

Adam really enjoys his morning at school. We have a quiet time together after lunch then he goes off with Lennie on bikes – I'm so glad his energy is returning.

Thursday 10 May
Adam has a huge breakfast, happy to be going to school. We worry when Vicki doesn't appear till 8:30 this evening; she missed her bus, managed to get half-way then *accepted a lift from a stranger*. Serious talks. She's begging for attention, isn't she. Feel incompetent again, determine to spread my attentions.

Friday 11 May
Think of all the things I'll be able to get done over the weekend, with no one here. Just about to leave for a flying visit to Grandad on my way to collect Adam from school when George phones: would I buy them food to take on the boat; they'll have to cook for themselves as their hosts unable to go. Oh, why don't I come along? Why indeed.

Grandad lucid for the first few minutes, then dizzy and sleepy. Talks a lot about music again. I'm interested as to why at this stage of his life music seems so much to the fore whereas it played no part previously; pure fantasy, it seems.

George returns, makes several transatlantic phone calls and takes us all out to the special seafood dinner; sticky, delicious.

Saturday 12 May
Drive Vicki to the station early, she's off for the weekend again. George, Adam and I get to the boat at 11:00 and nothing works. We sit there, bored, till batteries changed, points cleaned, etc. – about 1:30. Even then we can't make the fridge work.

Chug slowly along through frequent locks, rescue a baby duckling which was busy drowning in detergent at one of them. It spent the day in my anorak pocket and the night in a box with torn-up lavatory paper for bedding, water and chopped egg for supper. George disappears in search of a fish and chip shop, returns with a lovely Indian meal for us.

Sunday 13 May
Funeral at sea for duckling, which expired in the night.

We chug on a bit more, tie up and go for a walk. It was George's idea, but when I ask why he's galloping round so quickly he says every step is agony and he has to get back as fast as he can. I make us a salad lunch, we sunbathe a little then set off again, chug back a few locks before mooring for the night. They both sit and watch me prepare supper, then decide they aren't hungry; George decides he's ill and they both retire at 8:00.

Monday 14 May
Adam is most proficient at the locks as we chug slowly back. As soon as we arrive poor George forgets to duck and cracks his head against a doorway. We clean and tidy the boat, get home in time for a late lunch. Adam has enjoyed his weekend very much, although personally I feel I'd rather spend a weekend under a dripping tap than go through that again! George has many Dispirin, returns to London. Adam and I collect Vicki from the station and then the children and I sink thankfully into hot baths.

Tuesday 15 May
Joanne tells us her husband did well in the London Marathon: 3 hours 25 minutes, so we can start collecting the sponsorship money. Adam's blood count is low so he's down to half treatment.

We spend the rest of the day playing cards, Lego, snakes and ladders; it's a low-energy day but he's quite happy. Asks for boiled eggs for supper, then isn't sure he wants them. Tell him no one in the world has seen the inside of this egg; he thinks he knows what a boiled egg looks like, but does he? Is it set hard or just firm white with a runny yolk? Is the yolk pale yellow or almost orange? Will he see it when we slice the top off the egg or is it lower down? Will it just sit there, firm, or run over the egg cup? Get him interested enough to broach and eat two boiled eggs.

Wednesday 16 May
Take Adam to school, do a few jobs around the house and then it's time to pick him up, visiting Grandad en route.

We let the baby chicks out of the run for a while this afternoon — how we enjoy watching them, full of energy and curiosity yet so obedient to the calls of their mothers!

Thursday 17 May
A difficult day; Adam isn't up to going to school.

I know I should talk to someone, but I don't know who. Writing down my feelings helps a lot but there's no bounce-back. When I think about all the things I have to think about, it's hard to tell whether I'm being realistic or over-dramatic.

Maybe within marriage we always expect too much, perhaps we're doomed to disappointment in our husbands or wives. Perhaps that is why we feel a need for religion: craving everlasting acceptance and forgiveness.

Friday 18 May
School, go hold Grandad's hand, then Adam and I collect some sponsorship money around the village.

Saturday 19 May
Adam hardly moves from the sofa all day. I'm at my wits' end trying to amuse him gently, at the right level for the way he's feeling. George is in London househunting and feeling ill. My morale is round my ankles.

Sunday 20 May
George phones to ask if he can come to lunch, as he wants to see his father and has a visa application he'll help Vicki to complete. He wants to know what I *do* all day.

Spend ages on an extensive search for Victoria's birth certificate. Find it eventually, carefully filed under 'Receipts'. Sometimes my logic astounds me.

Monday 21 May
Adam to school, usual dreary routine. Must pull myself *out* of this downward spiral.

Tuesday 22 May
Adam had a bad dream and woke Vicki and me screaming, trotting round the house in a most distressed manner. Takes a long time to calm him; sit and stroke him back to sleep.

He's tense again this morning – it's vincristine day. Blood count up, so he's back on ¾ treatment. I ask Dr Morrison why they don't keep children on ¾ treatment once they have learnt that to put them up to full strength for two weeks knocks the white cell count so low they are then on no treatment or half treatment for the next few weeks. He says presumably it's all worked out by people who know what they are doing, then softens and says he'll ask Dr Evelyn if he has any literature on the logic behind it. Thank him: it does help if you can feel these things make sense.

Hear Katie is in the Westminster having her transplant; send her a card.

Wednesday 23 May
Adam feeling rough, aches and pains, much too tired to go to school, scratchy and on edge. He comes shopping with me because he wants new shoes; walks like a zombie.

He's feeling bloody-minded and wants to leave home. A difficult day.

Thursday 24 May
Sunny, and I promise to meet Adam from school at lunchtime with a picnic and we'll go straight to Birdland at Bourton-on-the-Water. He's keen. It's a beautiful drive. Adam tells me the trees and roadside flowers look so nice they make his heart go faster.

At Birdland he enjoys watching the Falkland penguins hopping about and swimming – their punk hairstyles look even stranger when wet. A large blue parrot follows us around saying Good boy, Good boy to Adam who gets embarrassed. We sit down with our picnic and cold drinks – suddenly we're dive-bombed by a squadron of emerald green parakeets! Flamingoes walking gingerly about on their fragile legs, caged birds everywhere, attractive gardens. We enjoy it.

We visit a trout farm on our way home – they're on to a good thing with that: not only do you pay to go in, you pay for the privilege of feeding their fish for them! It certainly has entertainment value though, the way the fish all boil up to the surface for the food. We've had a lovely afternoon out.

Friday 25 May
Adam too tired for school, just watches television. When I take Grandad his repaired watch, I find him vague, not so tearful. A friend of Vicki's comes this evening for one cockerel, six pullets – hope I sorted them out right! When George phones to say he'll be here on Monday, I tell him I bumped the front of the car and he isn't cross! Two swallows swooped, screaming, out of the garage on an apparent death mission just as I was pulling in; I jerked or ducked or something, just touched the edge of the garage doorway and the front of the car crumpled up. There's the merest splinter off the doorway, I can't understand it.

Saturday 26 May
A grey, cold and windy day, for which Adam curses the weather forecasters. I can't seem to get it across to him that they are the translators not the designers of our weather patterns.

We spend hours playing cards, board games; I try to will into him a feeling of security and love.

Sunday 27 May
Is there anything worse than a cold wet bank holiday weekend with everyone shut up together? Adam had another night of nightmares, is tired, achy, cross. We start another jigsaw puzzle. At midday I get so desperate I give Vicki some money and send her, Justin and Adam to the pub for a Coke and crisps before lunch – at least it's a change of scene for them.

The children spend the afternoon screaming at each other and me. Adam terribly uptight. The other two think I'm far too lenient with him, that I should make him do things instead of suggesting; that I should enforce an apology for rudeness rather than trying to ignore it. Explain to them that my only defence is to try my best to keep calm, that there are three television sets in the house just now and surely they can sort out their viewing without quarrelling. It seems natural to me that Adam should express his feelings of utter frustration sometimes. We are the natural recipients, it's because he loves us that he feels secure enough to express himself freely; he is in fact telling us he needs love, reassurance, more of a feeling of security. I wonder if they can begin to understand, or are they still too immature, in need of reassurance themselves?

I go upstairs. Adam comes into my room and hurls a chair at me. He's been packing his bag ready to leave home. Manage to get close enough to hug him – I can feel his tension – tell him I love him very much and ask what he thinks I can do to make him feel better. He doesn't know, but the physical contact obviously helps. We sit on the bed and hug each other, cry together. I can feel him beginning to relax as I stroke him.

I can't begin to express the feeling of absolute despair and failure this sort of day gives me. Peace and a degree of understanding were restored, but why did everything blow up like that in the first place? Why didn't I see it coming, stop it developing? Think it's only the release of writing all this down in the dead of night which holds me together at all.

No, there are still very happy times; the visit to Birdland the other day, the walk in the fields when I danced to the cattle; even today when I cuddled Adam better. Perhaps each day does have just enough that is positive to keep us going.

16

Monday 28 May
George appears for lunch, goes to visit his father, returns for a cup of tea and goes back to London.

I have a sore tooth.

Tuesday 29 May
Now the bank holiday is over and everyone's back at work, it's a lovely day. Pack up Vicki, Adam and Justin and take them to the Cotswold Park Farm Trust, a rare breeds survival place for farm animals. We like particularly the Highland Cattle, Strasbourg geese which look as though they've just had their feathers shampooed and can't do a thing with them, the Iron Age pigs. So many of the animals have appealing babies. We all enjoy the outing – till Adam says he's tired, it's time to go home.

During his bath we converse about where babies come from. I had told him it was a very special place in the mummy's tummy, so he wouldn't get it confused with the alimentary system; apparently he thought there was one special place for boy babies and another for girl babies and that you could choose. Try to clear that up, with a lot of simple words and an illustrated book.

Wednesday 30 May
Estimate for swallow-damage to car almost £300!

Grandad seems much better, but Matron makes a point of telling me he is still doing dreadful things.

Adam uptight again this evening – early bath – baths are relaxing and it does seem to calm him.

Thursday 31 May
Adam and Lennie go off on their bikes while I make soup and some cold dishes ready for lunch with Pauline. She wants to know why I don't simply tell George to come down more often.

Try to explain I don't just need George, I need him in a certain frame of mind and mostly he isn't in it. I know he suffers, for Adam and for his father, but he finds it easier to do it at a distance. She suggests I consult a good divorce lawyer, now.

Adam comes in, eats a good lunch with us, rushes off out.

Friday 1 June
It's wet and Adam is tired after yesterday's activities. George rings, says he'll be here for lunch on Sunday and how are things. Say wearily, Oh the same as usual – about a quarter of an inch the right side of intolerable, and he immediately tells me how busy he is. Someone has given him tickets to take Adam to the finals at Wimbledon – how nice of them.

Saturday 2 June
Sunny, and Adam is too. After lunch he keeps going out for little walks wearing his gorilla mask, but doesn't manage to frighten anyone. Shame.

Sunday 3 June
Early service. George arrives mid-morning, has a late breakfast and studies the housing section of the paper, then puts up Adam's new curtain poles.

After lunch I manage to find the opportunity to tell him I feel in need of a little rest and recuperation. Right, he says, how much money do you want? He suggests I take Adam to the south of France, to Ibiza or to Spain for the summer. Tell him, No, thank you, I don't want to do that, the Mediterranean countries are too conducive to tummy bugs and other odd little infections in the healthiest of us, so I don't think it would be right to take Adam there in his vulnerable state. He says the Med is only a couple of hours' flight away, I could take him for the whole summer, Adam enjoys that sort of holiday so much. Visions of commuting to Tuesday Clinics! Say again, Thank you, but no; could we maybe go to Disney World again for a couple of weeks, or to Denmark – Legoland and the Tivoli Gardens – the United States and Scandinavia are extremely hygienic, I'd feel safer, and would he come too? No, he won't contemplate it, both too far away, we'd never get medical insurance, he has no time, etc.

Well, Adam and I would both like to see Scotland. Right,

he has to go on business at the end of the month, if I can find someone to look after my livestock we can come too. He says he does feel guilty about my position, but he can't think of anything to do about it!

It isn't his fault either that I need emotional support or that he can't give it: just one of those things. He leaves, I cut grass, tears stinging.

Monday 4 June
Adam suddenly dissolves into tears when we arrive at school, neither of us know why. Calm again when we reach his classroom; think it better to leave him with smashing Mrs Wolf keeping an eye on him than to turn round and bring him straight home. Seems fine when I collect him, and has a good lunch. He's happily occupied afterwards when I take my hot tooth to the dentist.

The dentist X-rays it, taps it — I nearly go through the roof — *ow*. He says it's probably an abscess but he can fix it, I needn't lose the tooth. Sounds nasty, we're all jelly babies when it comes to toothache. He'll phone when he's studied the X-ray.

Tuesday 5 June
It's so cold Adam complains that his radiators aren't working! Get to Clinic early and give Joanne more sponsorship money — we've collected £181.80p round our little village.

Dr Morrison says exhaustive tests in the USA have shown it's better to put patients up to full strength treatment when the blood count allows, even if you know they'll have to go down again for a while, and Adam's back on full maintenance treatment for two weeks. When Adam is out of the room I ask if I could give him Valium when he gets into his screaming furious, throwing-things tempers; he says yes and again offers the service of their child psychologist, but I honestly don't think that would help.

Learn that Sheila died shortly after Joe, and Katie is seriously ill after her transplant which took place about ten days ago. Pray for them both.

Wednesday 6 June
When I arrive at the nursing home, Grandad has just had an accident all over the floor of the psychiatrics' sitting room, and

two of the girls take him to be cleaned up. I am given coffee in the staff sitting room, next door. They're a super bunch, dealing so cheerfully with him. One of the girls is nursing a bandaged hand; Kitty bit her, she says. I didn't know they had a cat – Oh no, Kitty is one of the old dears – the one with the *teeth*!

Grandad not at all with-it.

Adam full of energy, off on his bike with Lennie all afternoon. This village is ideal for him – it isn't on the way to anywhere, everyone knows him, and best of all the people seem to have such a caring and protective attitude, I'm quite happy to let him go off and exercise his independence. It's so good for him too – he's not nearly as shy now. People will stop me and tell me how polite and cheerful he is, how sensible on the roads on his bike, how the other kids gathered at the bus shelter were doing something silly but Adam wasn't; and, if someone spots him up to something they think I should know about, they tell me. Once when I wanted to go out and didn't know where he was to ask if he wanted to come too, all I had to do was walk a hundred yards and two or three people told me where he was, with whom, and what they were doing. Living here gives me a lovely feeling of security for him.

Thursday 7 June

Adam chose to spend all day at school today and went off with a packed lunch rather than miss morning school because of my dental appointment. The dentist drills hole up the back of my tooth, stuffs wire up hole, X-rays it, removes wire, gives me penicillin to take if it starts hurting and sends me home to drain for a week. Buy some mouthwash. Vicki wonders if my supper will end up in my sinuses, and the way that comment makes me snort with my mouth full, it may well!

Adam coped well with a full day at school, played rounders, fell over while playing 'rough games', tore his trousers and grazed his knee. I'm so glad he felt like playing rough games that I don't mind a bit about the torn trousers!

Vicki and Adam keep each other company while I go to another parents' evening at the JR with Martha and Maxine. It's informal – wine in plastic cups. The parents have apparently donated £1,500 towards this blood-typing machine, which can be bought in bits. More fund-raising events discussed. One drawback of village life: I'm reluctant to undertake jumble-sales etc. as I feel they all relate so sympathetically to us that it'd be nothing short of emotional blackmail.

I meet the mother of an 18 year old Briony talks of, who also has T-cell leukaemia, diagnosed two and a half years ago. He's doing all right on chemotherapy, goes to work although he has been very ill and gets pneumonia regularly. Two sets of parents whose children have been off treatment for 5 and 7 years respectively are there to give hope and encouragement to us all; several familiar faces at Clinic.

Friday 8 June
After his two very energetic days, Adam flakes out again. Not a particularly good day.

Saturday 9 June
Adam uptight, in need of a great deal of diplomacy, emotionally exhausting. He, Vicki and I have a picnic lunch in the garden, which lightens the mood somewhat.

Sunday 10 June
A beautiful day, Adam much better. Duncan rings and invites me to lunch on Tuesday. George arrives just before lunch, settles in the garden with newspapers. He fixes the new tractor drive-band for me, visits his father and goes back to London.

Tuesday 12 June
Ask Nick for a Valium prescription for Adam when he gets into his rages; he wants to know a lot of Adam's history and all about the rages. He knows I'm not a pill-pusher, and writes me up a few 2 mg. Valium for him when necessary. He also asks after Grandad, how I feel about Vicki's wanting to go to Australia, George and me. I understand her wanting to go away, I did at her age, I went to France. One tries to develop the best in one's children, help them to become well-balanced, capable, independent people. They need to go away from home in order to test things out – it's what parents have been striving for, they can hardly complain! I wish she'd chosen somewhere closer to home, but George is over there at least twice a year, he's met and approves Justin's parents, so it's all right with me. I feel I have to visit Grandad as frequently as I can, he

likes my visits and I'm the only person he has, apart from George, who isn't often here. As regards George and me, who knows.

Take Adam to lunch with Thea while I go on to Duncan's. He again says I should take a lover, I need the emotional comfort and support. Great, next time I go to the supermarket I'll pick up cat food, yoghurts, cheese and a nice lover, easy. Or should I advertise: one wife, second-hand, slightly shopsoiled, pear-shaped and grey-haired, takes two cigarettes to jump-start her lungs in the mornings? How would I organise the practicalities, anyway; bring him home and blindfold the children? The idea is at least a source of great personal amusement, but I think I'll have to settle for going to bed with a little light reading instead of a lot of heavy breathing.

Thea's sweet, says she'll have Adam any time I want to go and talk to Duncan or indeed do anything else(!). He's happy with her and laughs a lot at the little girls.

Wednesday 13 June
The dentist almost chokes me by making me laugh while he has both hands as well as various implements in my mouth. Tells me to come back in two weeks unless it hurts meanwhile. Now, does that comment inspire confidence or not?

Friday 15 June
Adam and I take the car in to be fixed, catch a bus and walk home, play games for the rest of the day. George appears unexpectedly at 6:30, says he has to go to a dinner at St Anne's College, where is it, would I find out while he changes, he'll be back here to sleep. Find map. Nick appears, give him a lager, show George where he's to go, see him off. Nick asks if the Valium is effective; explain I keep it for absolute emergencies and haven't yet used it. George returns very late and goes to bed leaving all the lights on.

Saturday 16 June
Adam seems to be building up to an explosion, says he won't ever be happy again and wants to kill all the bantams. He does calm down after I give him a Valium.

We all have lunch in the garden, spend a hilarious half-hour helping complete the accident claim-form for the car. Cause of accident, in driver's opinion: swallows, obviously, I insist. They screamed and dived straight at the windscreen. I lie sunbathing in my bikini and the children sprinkle breadcrumbs on my middle for the ducks and chicks, stand by with the camera. They are very funny, obviously tempted but don't quite dare to take it, thank goodness. George books a table for dinner, then takes the children shopping in Oxford. Happy.

Before we go out to dinner, we all race round the garden in a vain attempt to round up the bantams, which somehow puts us further into a light-hearted mood – we have a super evening out. Adam eats avocado then steak with enthusiasm. We're all relaxed – the day has turned out to be so enjoyable after an inauspicious start.

Sunday 17 June
Breakfast outside in the sun, newspapers escaping in the breeze, chicks and ducks shovelling up dropped crusts. I do petits poussins for lunch but don't manage to fool anyone into mistaking them for bantams!

After lunch, the children busy elsewhere, George and I sit on the grass by the pond and I ask him what are the advantages of our remaining 'married' – we seem to have all the disadvantages and none of the advantages. Why maintain such an uncomfortable status quo – maybe being free would give at least one of us a last chance. Nothing need change as regards the children; after all, he doesn't live at home with us now. I'd still do my best for his father, keep his mother's grave tidied, even do his laundry. I'm sorry we can't help each other more, but it doesn't feel right to me to go on trying to pretend – who are we trying to kid? I feel I should take independent advice.

He says do I want £10,000, would that make me feel more secure, I can always rely on him and I'm not to worry about money. I don't worry about money, that's not the point, I trust him absolutely as regards money – maybe having me entirely trusting and dependent on him is more of a drag than knowing where he stands and feeling free. He says that's very nice of me, he feels guilty about the children and maybe I need a psychiatrist rather than a lawyer. When I say I don't feel there is anything about me he likes or admires, he says I'm very good with the children. Nice to know I have something going for me.

During this conversation every flying, biting creature in the area lands on me and does its worst while George isn't bothered at all and he's right next to me. Must experiment with his after-shave.

Monday 18 June
Vicki comes home with stomach ache; give her sympathy, hot-water bottles, room service.

Tuesday 19 June
Very hot day, too good to spend in Clinic. When a doctor takes blood, gives vincristine, Adam almost faints. Jan has whooping cough, Dominic is very subdued, Katie we hear is a little better but it's still touch-and-go. Wouldn't go so far as Frankie, who says Clinic is an absolute shambles, but must remember to tell Maxine there was a whole spider's web across the front door when we got home! Adam off on his bike.

Wednesday 20 June
Visit Grandad while Adam's at school; he calls me Annette and says George brought him two orphans. Can't translate this. Keeps telling me he can't complain, although he seems to do little else. Manage to make him laugh.

Thursday 21 June
Drive three boys and a large picnic to the Aldershot Show where we all have a super day. All sorts of static exhibitions, things to look at, things to queue up and do, and a marvellous two-and-a-half-hour display in the arena. Stirring bands, horses, motor bikes, the paras with their free-fall drops – however do they gauge the landing so accurately! The Red Arrows were our favourites, they did such horrendous things you were certain they'd crash into each other – seem to miss by mere inches and zoom over us so low everyone ducks! The battle and rescue operations with helicopters are very exciting to watch. Such accuracy, everything so well-organised. I feel proud, and very British! We have a lovely day, then I manage to get us lost on the way home. On the way *home*, not even on the way *to* a place I'd never been to before . . .

Friday 22 June
George came back late last night and this morning we fly up to Edinburgh – a hot, uncomfortable flight, my ears popping all the time.

Beautiful countryside on our drive. We stop for lunch and shop for supplies.

We visit the Palace of Scone, where the Stone comes from; interior interesting but too ornate for my taste. The grounds are super, and they have pure white peacocks as well as the usual variety wandering around.

A little Japanese lady in traditional costume, who speaks no English but exhibits great personality, indicates with much bowing and tsk tsk noises that she wants us to stand together in front of the castle to be photographed. George thinks it's his beard which appeals. Is that the oddest thing about us? She gives us some Japanese coins and a strange little umbrella thing as souvenirs; Adam is utterly delighted with the whole episode!

Off to find the apartment George has borrowed. I make up beds for us all, unpack provisions; we wash, change and then have a super dinner in the hotel. This is Adam's sort of restaurant; he enjoys the food, the ambience, the bagpiper swirling through.

Saturday 23 June
We head off west, towards Loch Lomond, find it eventually. Countryside lovely; offer to do half the driving so George can look around, too, but he doesn't want me to. Sheep, cattle – only a very few Highland! – seagulls but hardly any other waterfowl around the lochs. We stop at a little pub for lunch; I ask for a bridie because I don't know what it is – turns out to be a sort of Cornish pastie with oatmeal instead of potato. The scenery around some of the smaller lochs further north much prettier than Loch Lomond, or perhaps we were on the wrong part of it.

We return to the flat, George starts going through his property ads again, complains about having missed one apartment, says he *must* be on the spot when something comes up. I ask why he doesn't take off a couple of weeks for serious house-hunting. He blows up, saying it doesn't happen like that, but while he's in London working he's so booked up with appointments it's days before he can find the opportunity to look at something which may be promising. It doesn't make sense to me: either he wants to make time for looking or he doesn't think it worthwhile. He clearly resents being here with us.

He manages to cheer up a bit and takes Adam for a swim in a beautiful hotel pool, after which we all go into town for an Indian supper. Adam likes the background music so much George makes a note of it and I later buy it for him: Lionel Ritchie, Can't Slow Down.

Sunday 24 June
Don't sleep until dawn. This all sounds lovely, and there are parts which are pure happiness I think for all of us, but the constraint between George and me becomes more clear. Leaden. Adam adores his father, we both need him, but I don't want him to spend time with us if he resents it and that is the feeling which comes across. Wonder what I should do. Feel I should rationalise the situation. Can't go in 'off the street' to see a solicitor, don't want to embarrass George by going to someone we both know, can't really go round asking people if they know a good divorce lawyer. Everything seems intolerable, as things tend to do in the middle of the night. My current favourite prayer is:

> Please God grant me the strength to change those things which I ought to change;
> The serenity to accept those things which I cannot change;
> And the wisdom to know the difference.

We lunch with some friends of George, then spend a few hours in or around the swimming pool at the hotel, have a light supper there. George talks again about my taking Adam away for the summer, perhaps to a friend's villa in Minorca, but couldn't come with us and vetoes the idea of going anywhere more hygienic even when I remind him how horribly ill he and Angela were in Ibiza once.

To bed, exhausted enough to sleep after a couple of hours' turmoil. At least we both react to Adam in a manner which I think prevents him from feeling there's anything wrong; we both project such gentle loving concern I'm sure he doesn't suspect.

Monday 25 June
George phones a couple of London estate agents and tells me there are two or three likely riverside properties but they'll be sold tomorrow without his having had a chance to see them and there'll be nothing else for two or three years, it's imperative he be on the spot.

What he considers important in life and what I consider important seem to be creeping further and further apart. How *can* one make such a basic mistake as to marry the wrong person? No, I can't think that, there have been very good times.

I suggest going to see Edinburgh Castle today, think there may be suits of armour, Scots Guards, canon, various things of that sort to interest Adam. George doesn't think it would be interesting at all; he wants to go to Loch Ness – so we head up to Loch Ness.

Lovely lovely countryside, fantastic mountains and glens, once more the scenery around the smaller, previously unheard-of lochs much more interesting than the famous one. Tease Adam that he mustn't catch the Loch Ness Monster: I wouldn't know how to cook it. Rocky outcrops containing a lot of quartz, chunks of grey and rose striped rock, or sparkly white; Adam even finds sparkly silver and gold pieces – we treasure-hunt, come back with a bagful.

Tuesday 26 June
George takes Adam for a last swim while I pack up, sort out beds, clean bathrooms and kitchen, we have brunch and set off on our way home. A vastly superior flight to the one up, although my ears still hurt. I don't travel well. Good to get home again.

17

Wednesday 27 June
Adam wakes early, rushes out to see to the chicks and ducks – ducks all right but he can only find two bantams and a lot of feathers under the medlar tree. We're all very upset, then find Little Black Bantam stoically sitting on 11 eggs under the hedge. Carefully move her and the eggs into the safety of the chick house.

I visit Grandad. His 'lost' words seem to be replaced by 'boats' today instead of 'music'. The doctor gave him some boats for his foot but they weren't doing him any good; he had some nice boats for lunch yesterday. I took him chocolates, he says, Thank you, would you like to share the boats?

Thursday 28 June
Little Black Bantam didn't appreciate having her eggs moved to safety, she's let them go cold and Adam is very upset. He seems fit though and goes happily to school while I have final session at the dentist's.

Write to Tom in Cardiff asking if he can recommend a good lawyer in the matrimonial causes sphere in this area. Think our few days in Scotland proved our marriage just doesn't exist, it's an intolerable farce and it would be sensible for me to try to put my position in order. If I can find someone through Tom, asking for advice won't be so embarrassing.

After lunch Adam needs cuddling and is still rather upset about the cold eggs, so we spend the afternoon reminiscing about our feathered friends.

Last year, we were keen to have baby ducklings, but as we had inadvertently ended up with too many drakes and not enough ducks, they were enjoying their sex lives far too much to take 28 days off sitting on eggs. They buried eggs in clutches under straw in the duck house but positively refused to sit on them. We borrowed from friends a broody hen and a bantam – not having bantams of our own then – and installed them in the maternity units in the back of the duck house, shut in for the first 24 hours, then with daytime access to a small enclosure.

On the second day the bantam wanders out to stretch her legs and can't find her way back in, panics. I try to guide her, she panics further, flies over the wire-netting and disappears through the hedge at the bottom of the orchard into a field full of bullocks and mud. I squeeze through after her, with visions of Someone Else's Bantam disappearing forever into the sunset, and spend a jolly hour galumphing about amid curious bullocks and evil-smelling mud which seems determined to cling onto my Wellies, trying to creep close enough to toss my anorak over her. Manage in the end, return her to her eggs which she greets with delight – obviously thought she'd never see them again. She sat on them hard, without budging, till 9 hatched.

The speckled hen, on the other hand, sat peacefully on her foster-eggs for more than two weeks, then we had such a beautiful day she decided it was far too nice to spend it inside, and I found her contentedly doing a little gardening. She thought the seedling lettuce too untidy and inhibited access to Interesting Insects, so she was cleaning them out for me, with a great show of industry and little disapproving noises in the back of her throat. No way could she be persuaded to return to maternal duties, having Tasted Freedom; she was ignominiously despatched home in a grocery carton.

We did our best with the eggs in a contraption warmed by a lamp, spraying and turning them several times daily, but it didn't work. I had heard an egg can be hatched if you keep it in your cleavage, but unfortunately I wasn't endowed with one of those.

Adam loves these remember-when stories, they seem to help him accept the vagaries of ducks and bantams; he feels better about Little Black Bantam's deciding not to continue sitting on her eggs.

Friday 29 June
Take Adam to school, shop, unshop, visit Grandad. Adam comes down to the Church with me this afternoon, we take fresh roses to Granny. When it's my turn to clean the Church, Adam comes along full of enthusiasm which rapidly decreases

when I won't allow him to do what he considers the interesting parts – 'testing' the bells and the organ, finding a ladder so he could clean the stained-glass windows. He whips around with spray-polish and then slopes off to the little shop for crisps.

Ted calls to borrow the baby tractor, asks how things are. Tell him I'm contemplating divorce. He says he's very sorry to hear the situation is like that and to go cry on his shoulder whenever I want to; could he tell Briony or would I rather he didn't? Say of course he can, although no one else knows, except Nick probably guessed the way things were heading.

Saturday 30 June
Adam and I do some gardening and enjoy it. Vicki spends the entire day tidying her room. Adam shunts a great deal of rubbish up to the orchard with the baby tractor and trailer – he likes that sort of job very much, so it stimulates me into rubbish-production in the garden! A happy day. George phones to say he'll be back tonight.

When he comes I tell him I've written to ask Tom to recommend a solicitor. He asks why, and when I tell him I don't want to approach anyone we know, says it's very nice of me. Asks if I told Tom why I wanted a solicitor; say, Of course: matrimonial.

Sunday 1 July
Awake early enough but feel I can't go to communion: I'm not in the right frame of mind. I hurt, my heart is pounding, I feel like an accident looking for somewhere to happen. My stomach gripes so much I can't even finish lunch; retire and leave Vicki to serve the rest after soup, but then Adam gets upset so I reappear to comfort him.

George works on papers all afternoon. When I make him tea – the children aren't around – he laughs, Well, are you going to sue me for divorce this week. I just dissolve into tears and he can't understand at all. He asks how much money I want to give me the independence to do as I please; tell him what I want is a more peaceful frame of mind; money doesn't come into it. That we keep expecting things of each other which don't come about so we disappoint each other and it hurts too much; maybe if we were divorced we wouldn't expect so much. He says again he thinks what I need is a good psychiatrist; that he knows I take a lot of strain but that he helps all he can. If I do see a lawyer, I'm to ask George personally for anything I want, not to make the mistake of having someone else ask on my behalf; I can have anything I want, within reason. He can't see that this is just what I can't have.

Vicki goes up to London with him.

Monday 2 July
Wake very early. Adam feels off-colour and doesn't go to school. We collect Vicki and Justin from the station. Martha the paediatric social worker phones to say Katie died a week ago. Write to her parents, feeling desperately sorry for them, yet trying to feel pleased that we've decided not to subject Adam to transplantation.

Tuesday 3 July
A quick Clinic and we return to find Vicki and Justin securing the strawberry netting, watering the garden. We all do some gardening after lunch, have a bonfire later, cut the orchard, and I begin to think perhaps I can return to some sort of normal pattern; I don't hurt as much as yesterday.

Wednesday 4 July
Take Adam to school, wash floors and do other similarly-uninteresting things. Visit Grandad. He looks fit but doesn't manage one coherent sentence. Matron tells me he's on antibiotics for a foot infection.

Ted calls to borrow the strimmer and talks to me beautifully. It's a lovely warm feeling, knowing he's keeping an eye on me by borrowing things!

Adam goes down to Viv to have his hair cut, comes back in great excitement to tell me we can have one of Dennis' cockerels. I offer to pay young Dennis for him, he refuses charmingly, and they deliver one vocal cockerel shortly, happy to find him a good home. Adam has been absolutely super recently, responsive and such a joy to have around.

Thursday 5 July
Adam to school, but distinctly off when I collect him at 12:15.
After lunch I feel it imperative to leave him watching

television while I go over to see Ted. Tell him I think I need some sort of help, does he think I need a psychiatrist, as George suggests; am I going mad? He agrees I need help, but thinks my reactions are perfectly normal, therefore I need some sort of expert counselling service rather than a psychiatrist. He doesn't think I am neurotic – that's such a relief. May he speak to Briony and Nick in order to find someone they think I could relate to easily – he won't if I'd rather not. Of course he can: I came to him in the first place because somehow I couldn't summon up the courage to make and then keep an appointment with Nick not because I couldn't talk to him. Remembering what he's said to me, I could have rung Nick direct; don't know why I didn't have the nerve.

Ted thinks I am too bound up with Adam to the detriment of my own life, but has to agree it's natural in the circumstances. I'm perfectly happy to have him discuss me with Briony and Nick, so grateful to have him as an easily-available intermediary. He's a lovely sympathetic sensible man, I'm so glad I know him. He hugs me beautifully as I go and that alone helps a lot. Feel so much better simply for having shared my feelings with him.

Adam and I walk down to Phil's. Their garden, house, pool, are lovely, immaculate. Adam and Phil swim, the water is 85°; we lounge around the pool on beautiful garden furniture with lovely cold drinks and watch wild baby rabbits playing on the lawn – they're enchanting and Linda says they don't even damage their seedlings. Then a barbecue. Adam eats a tremendous amount and we're outside till after 10:00 – a super evening.

Friday 6 July
Adam too tired for school after his swimming, and massive intake of food and late night.

Visit Grandad who is on bed rest after falling and giving himself a black eye and cut head. Tells me his foot tickles, or is it his shoulder, something does but he isn't sure what.

Ted phones after lunch and asks me to go over for coffee. He says Nick, Briony and he have discussed things and suggest I should see a psychotherapist who lives nearby. Nick will come and see me to fix an appointment; he thinks I should see this man two or three times a week. Again he hugs me as I leave – I think that is far more beneficial than spending hours with a psychotherapist would be, but can't really say so!

Tom rings and offers to come and see me himself if that would help – isn't that lovely, all the way from Bath. Tell him many thanks but no, I think it is better to keep things a step apart, although I greatly appreciate his kindness.

Saturday 7 July

Another scorching sunny day. We tidy Granny's grave then sit out in the sun for a while, playing cards. Adam helps me pick strawberries later, laughs at me as we both try to pick my toe-nails among the strawberry leaves – shouldn't wear nail polish in the strawberry bed! We remember how Sheba used to enjoy lying alongside the netting and sucking strawberries through.

George phones to say he won't be here tonight after all but will come 9:00-ish in the morning to collect Adam and take him to Wimbledon. Adam is very disappointed and convinced George will phone tomorrow to say he's still too busy to come for him. Cuddles, reassurance.

Sunday 8 July

George here before 9:30, Adam quiet and tense waiting for him, cheers up when he arrives. Make breakfast for George, pack them up a nice lunch to take, give them my camera, plenty of cold drinks, cushions; the car is loaded up, we call goodbyes, Vicki slams George's door shut – and the window disappears down inside the door. Catastrophe. Right, says George, we can't go, can't leave a car unlocked in London, that's it. Adam's lower lip trembles. Tell George how lucky he is, he can take my car. He's reluctant to do that as he knows I'm supposed to be meeting Tom and family. Finally persuade him to take Adam off in my car and leave me his keys. I'll do a practice run around the village and if I decide I can manage his car I can still go. He doesn't for a moment believe I'll drive his car, can't believe I don't mind if my lunch date has to be postponed anyway – Wimbledon can't be, after all. Eventually we transfer car contents and wave them off.

Do practice run in the Jaguar and decide that with a clean windscreen and a fair wind I could manage it. Vicki's most impressed, she didn't think I'd dare, either. Perhaps I'm beginning to branch out.

Lovely lunch and afternoon with Tom and co., home about 7:00 with the name and address of a lawyer in Oxford, recommended by Tom.

George and Adam beat me to it. They, Vicki, Justin and I then spend the next couple of hours dismantling the door of the Jaguar in order to locate and reposition the window. This is difficult but we manage eventually to get it in the closed position which at least means he can park it with confidence.

George stays to supper, talks Australia pleasantly to Vicki and Justin, asks if Tom gave me the advice I wanted. Explain again that all I asked of him was the name and address of a good divorce lawyer near here, which he gave me; don't want to involve friends more than that. He seems pleased.

Tell him Ted thinks I should see a psychotherapist who is in private practice, would that be all right. He grunts, Oh well, if we have to pay for what you need we have to pay for it, but if Nick also thinks it necessary surely BUPA will cover it. I've never seen George's BUPA policy, so I don't know. George then says he's going to put in an offer of an extortionate amount for a house he likes. The very figure makes my blood run cold. Priorities, priorities.

He asks Chris to waterproof the leaking fishpond and to redo Adam's bathroom. Adam is very pleased about both these things. He's had a lovely day with his father and is sleepy now.

Monday 9 July

Peter comes round to start cleaning out the fishpond and Adam helps him. They have a lovely time and put rescued creatures into the large paddling pool – frogs, newts – including greater crested newts, which are an endangered species now – and amazingly around 30 goldfish are transferred into the temporary accommodation. Adam happy – this is the sort of project a boy can really put his heart into – and comes back inside with black sticky mud everywhere, including ears, eyes, nose. Lengthy scrub down in the bath and we even need fresh rinsing water.

Try to work out what I could achieve from psychotherapy: to expand my mind without blowing it; to be able to see clearly whether George and I could get closer or whether it'd be better to finalise our marriage so he could perhaps find someone else who could give him more than I can; what effect such a break would have on Adam, Vicki, George and me.

Tuesday 10 July
Clinic. Dr Evelyn says we must get away for a holiday, we need a break. Oh gee. Adam's blood count is still low, half treatment again.

Wednesday 11 July
Adam to school, then I take a big bowl of strawberries in to the nursing home, hope there will be enough for all the people who use the psychiatrics' sitting room. Sister says thank you, yes, plenty, and do I take chocolate in for Grandad? Yes, just a bar or so at a time. Could I bring diabetic chocolate in future, he's all right but he will keep feeding it to diabetics. Agree. Tell Grandad I've brought strawberries for them all and hope he enjoys them; he says George brought him one yesterday morning and another in the afternoon, it was very interesting so he was all right. He says he went for a drive with my father (who died 14 years ago) yesterday but it was so snowy they didn't go far. The music is good today. How am I? His legs hurt him, Oh the pain, the pain.

Collect Adam from school. He's been doing a French project, they had a French breakfast of rolls, coffee and something he calls crabs. Judicious questioning reveals this to be croissants rather than seafood.

Vicki and Justin in Oxford yet again. Adam and I lunch together, then Lennie appears and they play swingball. So I summon up the courage to ring and make an appointment with the lawyer. Nick phones to say he hoped to look in yesterday or today but has been very busy, and then he dries up, so I tell him Ted told me they'd discussed things and thought they'd found a psychotherapist I should see. He seems vastly relieved, says he's spoken to him but would like to discuss things face to face with me, so I make an appointment to go to the Health Centre to see him. I've more courage now I've set a few wheels in motion.

Thursday 12 July
Take Adam to school, Vicki and Justin for their bus to Oxford, then go to the Health Centre to see Nick. Explain I feel

ashamed about asking for help, feel I should be able to manage everything, not just the sunny side of life. He says I'm not to feel that, he thinks I've taken a bundle in the last few months, and that everyone needs help at some time in their lives; he thinks I need to be able to talk things out with someone, and would I feel free to call on him or go over to see Ted at any time, particularly when this psychotherapist is away. I have a sudden feeling he thinks I'm in a worse state than I really am; thank him and tell him I am not suicidal, I have too strong a sense of obligation and also too much curiosity. He seems a little taken aback but I'm sure that's what he was thinking. He reiterates, call any time I want to. It gives me a lovely warm feeling.

Collect Adam and go up to see his work. His writing is very neat but the French phrases do not match the translations.

Later, while Mr Burrett helps Adam mend a puncture, I go over to see Ted, tell him I've seen Nick. I wanted to thank him too and also to reassure him that I am not suicidal. He said, Thank you for telling me, I was worried, and hugs me. Whatever is happening to me, My God, they really did think . . .

George phones at 8:00, says he had a message at 11:00 saying phone home urgently, what is it? Don't know, it must have been Vicki, who isn't here, it certainly wasn't me. Can't stop myself from saying, Gee thanks, I appreciate your sense of urgency especially in the circumstances. He produces all sorts of problems about seeing Vicki and Justin in London tomorrow and when I say I'll take them he gets abusive. He lost both the houses he offered for so I guess I should be understanding.

Friday 13 July

Drop Adam at school, Vicki and Justin at the station, take Grandad cheese biscuits because I've forgotten to buy diabetic chocolate. He's awake, dribbly, vocal but not making any sense, wants to give me tablets. Tell him I have everything I need, thank you. Ask if he enjoyed the strawberries I took along the other day. Oh yes, strawberries, very interesting, George brought him one. Hold his hand for about 40 minutes then go collect Adam from school.

After lunch Adam watches a film on television, I curl up

next to him. The psychotherapist phones: he can see me on Thursday afternoon but I can't take Adam with me.

George arrives about 8:00 with Vicki and Justin – they collected their air tickets and he gave them a nice lunch out. George rather tense and withdrawn, feeling vindictive about having lost both the properties he offered for, talking wild retribution. He thaws a little over supper.

Saturday 14 July
Vicki and Justin disappear into Oxford early; George difficult all morning. Says, Well, tell Vicki I hope she has a good time in Australia and ask her what she is going to use for money; if I'd realised she was going into Oxford this morning I wouldn't have come down – lots of that sort of thing. He finds two tins of black shoe polish with a little in each, plays hell because I don't have enough polish for him to clean his shoes. I walk down to the little shop – why *me* not him – but they've run out of black, too.

He's so prickly I say, I wish I could help you George, and he says, No one can help me but never mind I may drop dead from a heart attack. So may I, I suppose; is that meant to be a comforting thought? The more tense and cross he becomes, the calmer and more reasonable I get – it must be infuriating. I say, Why do you feel you have to say that to me? Oh, it'd solve a lot of problems and I wouldn't have the worries and frustrations I have now, he says. I think he needs help more than I do. He has a headache and is absolutely impossible until lunch. I make tandoori chicken, rice, salad and poppadums; he feels better. Goes off to visit his father briefly and returns to accompany Adam and me to young Tracey's wedding. Adam is very excited, he hasn't been to a wedding before.

Chris and his daughter arrive at the Church in a cart decked with ribbons and flowers and bridesmaids, pulled by two beautiful shire horses, coats and brasses shining, coachman smartly liveried. It's a lovely service, the bride and bridesmaids so pretty, the most delightful wedding I've ever been to. (And that includes Zoe's, when I caught the two smallest bridesmaids halfway up the sweeping curve of the staircase, tugging up their long dresses, flower-coronetted heads together as they compared tummy-buttons . . .)

Adam is invited to join the bride, groom and bridesmaids

on the cart – he is rather embarrassed but thrilled! George stays at the reception for half an hour and then goes off to a garden party in Hertfordshire. Adam and I stay on, we're enjoying it very much.

Vicki is convinced George said he'd come back for them on Wednesday night and take them on to Gatwick on Thursday morning from here. She's upset he now says he wants them to spend the night in his London flat on Wednesday but doesn't know what his commitments are and may not be able to see them. Try to explain a night in London would be more sensible, taking the geography into account, and that he was lashing out because he was hurt, under strain; try to cement the communication gap a little.

Sunday 15 July

Go to early communion, leaving all the children here. Later, we take Vicki and Justin to his grandparents in Gerrards Cross. On our return we pick more strawberries and Adam delivers bowlsful to neighbours. I get something in my eye; it hurts a lot but I can't see anything there. Lid over lid, eye bath, don't do anything. Eye a furious red and hurting. Decide I need help but can't drive anywhere. If I go to a neighbour it would seem sensible to go to Ted and Briony, the doctors, rather than to anyone else. There are so many cars in their drive I don't; go back in to sit and think. Brain wave: peel and chop an onion until I have cried the foreign body into the corner of my eye! Remove a seed of barley genre with a sharp spike on each end of it; no wonder it hurt. Am immensely pleased with myself for managing this on my own. Once upon a time, I'd thought Independence is, your very own drain rods. Now maybe I should revise that to Independence is, knowing how to get something out of your own eye. Perhaps this time I have made a medical breakthrough!

I'm still in a muddle about what exactly I hope to gain from (a) the lawyer I'm seeing on Tuesday and (b) the psychotherapist I'm seeing on Thursday. And what to do with Adam while I see them.

Monday 16 July

Same jolly routine – take Adam to school, shop, go see Grandad – who seems to be failing. He turns white and faint if they try to get him up, feels very cold to the touch. Complains about pain in his legs, at least he thinks it's his legs, it may be his eyes. Asks about Mother, how is she, and with a flash of inspiration I say, Oh, the same as ever (Quite good, that, I think: after all once dead there you are). He talks absolute nonsense, holds and strokes my hand. I would be only too pleased to feel I could stop visiting him, but he obviously appreciates my visits so I must continue to go as often as I can.

Adam is happily helping Peter with the fishpond, has a super day. He keeps bringing in 'creatures' captured in a coffee jar; we look them up, try to identify and find out about them.

Tuesday 17 July

Lose Adam while I'm cooking his breakfast. He went to let the ducks out and I find him just standing in the orchard. Nothing's the matter, he just wants to stand, look and listen. Absorb things. Little, important things. After about half an hour he comes in, eats breakfast. He cries silently all the way to Clinic, can't explain what has upset him and the silence of his distress is terrible. To make matters worse we had forgotten it is vincristine week, go up to Joanne in haematology for the blood sample and then he has to have the IV downstairs later. Dr Keith manages first time, thank goodness. Martha comes over to talk but Adam doesn't respond. Blood count slightly improved so he's up to ¾ treatment, back next week.

After lunch Adam stays here helping Peter with the pond while I go back into Oxford to see the lawyer about separation or divorce. He thinks legal separation just now, and gives me a list of questions to ask George.

Adam and I drive to Gerrards Cross to collect Vicki and Justin. On the way back as someone streaks past me on the motorway I say, I'm doing 70, I wonder what he's doing. Adam immediately says, Speeding, which sets us all in a mood of general gaiety.

We have a celebration supper, a good evening. Vicki and Justin sit like two of the wise monkeys with their arms around each other, eyes shiny with excitement. I can't really believe that tomorrow they're off to the other side of the world.

18

Wednesday 18 July
An odd sort of day, waiting for it to be time to take Vicki and Justin to the station. Adam didn't go to school but puts a lot of energy into helping Peter. Vicki and Justin decide to go into Oxford one last time; I visit Grandad, then take Mrs Burrett to visit newly tonsil-less grandchild. On their return Vicki and Justin, in a state of excited suspense, half-watch television.

At last it's time to go to the station – we get there a little early and then no one can think of anything sensible to say. We repeat the usual inanities as people do in such a situation, then Vicki and Justin kiss us goodbye twice each and insist we go, while we're all still laughing.

We can't persuade the chicks to bed which upsets Adam. He says his head aches – it is thundery – so give him a Valium and then a nice relaxing bath. Says he isn't sure he'll feel well enough to picnic at the Wildlife Park with his class tomorrow.

Thursday 19 July
Still awake well past midnight when I realise (a) Chris's dogs are barking loudly and (b) the chicks are out, so I flit around the garden in my nightie making sure there's no fox about. Back in bed, think how silly to go out like that: it could have been The Fox, not a fox. The newspapers have been full of stories of a terrorist rapist in the Leighton Buzzard area who does terrible things to his victims and police say will probably Strike Again.

Adam does go to school with a picnic. I whirl around doing chores and it's 3:15 and he's home again before I know it – they dropped him off on their way through. He's had a good day, drinks down three glasses of lime juice and rushes into the garden to help Peter; I leave him with instructions to go back with Peter and stay with Willow if I'm not back when they finish work.

It seems a forbidding prospect, to see a perfect stranger and start trying to tell him everything about us, but somehow it happens quite naturally. He says very little; I talk, I cry, I come out like jelly – an extraordinary experience.

Psychotherapist said keeping a diary is a good idea to release my feelings but I should be able to express them to another person and get feed-back. Yes, I know that, but my feelings at the moment seem too ambivalent to express adequately anyway.

Friday 20 July
Adam comes shopping with me, we buy him new jeans and he's very pleased. I visit Grandad on our way home – Adam stays in the car – and find him sitting on the bed stark naked, looking at the newspaper. He says he feels cold, and can't find the carrots. I help him into some pyjamas, he starts taking them off again, says he needs a coat on, he's so cold. Tell him I'm not surprised he's cold, sitting around with no clothes on, and why doesn't he get back into bed and stay there today. Oh, that's a good idea, Katherine, I never thought of that, he says, and climbs meekly back into bed.

Saturday 21 July
Do the chores while Adam watches Saturday morning television. George rings to say he has nothing else to do so he'll be out here for lunch if that's all right. The Last Resort.

Tell George I've seen the lawyer, explain the things he wants to know and ask him to make contact. He seems to find the whole thing funny for some reason.

Sunday 22 July
I dreamed Adam was bleeding from the bowel and woke in a cold sweat in his doorway.

I think telling George I've seen a lawyer and the counsellor has taken a lot of the heat out of our relationship – it's been the best weekend for a long time. Maybe he's been hoping for ages I'd ask him for a divorce, too polite to mention it himself? Anyway, he flits around finding things to fix, getting Adam to help him with odd jobs, being a fully-integrated member of the family, relaxed and cheerful. He sees Chris about redoing Adam's bathroom – Adam's pleased at the idea of a new bath which won't sandpaper his bottom. He goes to visit his father;

agrees with Adam that we could construct a waterfall into the fishpond, talks about pumps. A buoyant weekend.

Monday 23 July
Still feel good about the weekend. Taking positive action has done a lot for me as well as George. I wonder why exactly the same situation can be intolerable for me and then somehow acceptable. It can't always be put down to hormone levels.

Adam comes shopping with me, not too subdued after his active weekend. He stays in the car while I visit Grandad, who is asleep when I arrive. Calls me Alice when he wakes, says at first he thought I was Katherine. Surprised when I tell him I *am* Katherine. Seems to think he's had an operation, talks a lot of nonsense, very disorientated, crying, hanging on to me, not wanting me to leave him. Most distressing.

Adam plays swingball, goes off on his bike, generally spends an outdoor, extrovert afternoon and evening.

Tuesday 24 July
Clinic. Out quite quickly, back next week. Dr Morrison says it's a horrendous Clinic next week and jokes he's planning to be off sick – I'd better remember to get there early! Adam still on ¾ treatment.

He yawns a lot today – laughs a lot too, but wants to be quiet with me rather than outside playing with Lennie. We play various games, read, cuddle, tease each other. He drapes his imitation snake several times in such well-chosen places that each time I inadvertently come across it, it makes me jump and yelp, leaving Adam weak with laughter at his stupid mother, and enjoying such a sense of superiority!

He notices the sunset with absolute delight this evening – it's orange, purple, pink and blue, decorated with little white clouds like fluffy cottonwool balls. I love that child so much.

We clear away lamps, ornaments, before we go to bed, ready for the carpet cleaner tomorrow.

Wednesday 25 July
Two cards from Vicki en route to Hong Kong: in the first she's excited; the second, just out of Bahrain, she's tired and missing us, which doesn't exactly inspire confidence.

Lennie arrives before breakfast, he and Adam disappear

into the roof of the garage. I yell at them, Come down, you *know* you aren't allowed to climb over the car and go up there. Not very tactful of me. Lennie leaves, Adam arms himself with my kitchen knife, locks me out of the house and yells for my blood. He *hates* me.

I pick some sweet peas, ignoring the situation. There becomes little point in defending an unassailed citadel, after all. He emerges in a while, still very wound up and abusive. I talk gently and calmly, manage to disarm him, hug him; we both go back into the house. Thank heavens the carpet cleaner is late. Valium with breakfast.

Adam engrossed in watching the carpet cleaner so I shoot off for a quick visit to Grandad, who has wet his bed and is busy turning out all his drawers, wearing only a pyjama jacket. Fetch someone to sort him out.

Matron tells me he's very confused now, as well as being doubly incontinent. He gets everything in his room in such a state and stuffs the most unlikely objects into his commode, so would I bring a suitcase in and take everything home, leaving him only his pyjamas and a cardigan?

She says he's fading away and if he gets an infection which would carry him off it would be wrong to strive to prolong his life. He is spoonfed something like strained baby-food for lunch, followed by custard. Clings to my hand, seems pleased with the sweet peas and chocolate I took.

Go home, feeling shaky, make Adam lunch. He disappears off on his bike for the afternoon, full of energy. The noise of the steam cleaner is deafening.

What is the common denominator in all this and why do I feel so sore? Worry is not only non-productive, it's destructive. Sometimes I seem to catch a glimpse of something, a clarity like the sky on a clear frosty night, during which there does seem to be a meaning, a logic, in life. Then it's all gone again in an instant, I relapse once more into a thick humid mist like warm soup, cursing my inability to express the clarity when it appears, to pin it down with words which would perhaps give it a form I could hang on to.

Thursday 26 July
Adam tired today, having played so hard yesterday. Lennie appears twice; I send him away at Adam's request. We picnic

in the garden at lunchtime, laze around on a rug watching the chicks and ducks, gazing into the pool, talking. Dragonflies dart about like miniature helicopters, big green ones and little bright blue ones. Lie on our tummies and part a few blades of grass: there's a whole new world. It's 'time out' and very precious. He drives the tractor a little, helps me do a few gardening jobs, very lazily, with the robin keeping us company.

Friday 27 July
Up early and talk to Vic about the new bathroom. Adam comes with me to bring back Grandad's things. He's asleep when we arrive, and when he wakes he tries to eat his chocolate through the wrapping – Adam helps him most sympathetically. I tell him we're taking his clothes to be cleaned, but he doesn't seem to notice what I'm doing anyway. Wash the chocolate off him. At least he's in bed, doesn't say or do anything to frighten Adam. He goes to sleep again, so we leave. Adam says later, Poor Grandad, I hope he'll soon be dead. Silently echo these sentiments.

We wander about trying to find places for things – with George's, his mother's and now his father's things around as well as ours, this little house is full to overflowing.

Saturday 28 July
I don't know why I visit George's father so often. He hardly seems like a person now. I don't go to witness his degradation – it isn't humiliation because he isn't aware of it – and he leaves me feeling physically ill. I'm not masochistic, I don't go in order to chalk up Brownie points in heaven, I know I don't go with love, so why? I have a conscience, think he needs someone, and he really has no one else; is that a good enough reason for what it does to me?

George rings to say he has nothing to do and can he come down. Of course. He's here before lunch, finds jobs to do without my even hinting. He chops large chunks off the plum tree which darkens the kitchen; Adam helps load the pieces onto the trailer, drives the tractor up to the orchard.

It's too hot to go to the Traction Engine Rally; we loll about in the garden, Adam and I playing cards, George reading his papers. George later barbecues supper for us. A good day.

George has made a courtesy call to my solicitor and shows

me a letter he proposes to send. Am interested to see I'd under-estimated his earnings by more than two-thirds; he earns an immoral amount, but then he works extraordinarily long hours. I would like George himself to propose financial arrangements for me and the children.

Sunday 29 July
Wake at 3:45, again at 4:45, 5:45, so give in and go to the early service.

Another beautiful day which we spend outside after George and Adam have visited Grandad and brought back the television set and the rest of his clothes.

Adam quiet and yawning, but can't help thinking even when he's sleepy he is still enjoying life, whereas the two children who had transplants aren't. In one way I want to smother him with treats, buy him the moon; in another way want to keep life as 'normal' as possible. Most parents who lose a child suffer sudden bereavement as a result of an accident, or lose a very sick child who has suffered for months in hospital. We have a chance to make the most of a fairly normal life, and at the same time have been given a very strong warning, notice to prepare. It's still a puzzle. Someone with a 99% chance of survival could still be the one to die; they say Adam has only around five or ten percent chance of surviving so we try to become accustomed to the idea of his dying yet he could be the unexpected chap who makes it.

I hope whenever he does die I'll still be around to help him do it nicely, and that he won't linger like Grandad.

George says he'll take Adam away in a boat later in August and that I can take him away fairly soon. Tells me to order new tractor engine, new bathroom equipment. I feel he's doing his best to put my house in order for me, and love him for that. He's doing what he feels to be important, to the best of his ability.

Monday 30 July
Phone Pauline and ask if I could take Adam to her house at Milford for a few days; she'll check and let me know.

Adam dozy, not doing very much at all. Thank heavens yet again for television.

Tuesday 31 July
Clinic. Adam's count is down, so ½ treatment for two weeks. When Dr Morrison asks how he is and I tell him not a lot of energy or appetite he says, Okay, that's as maybe, but I've two children up on the Ward just now who look a lot worse. He then apologises and says he guesses that isn't a great deal of comfort. He's right, it isn't; I can tell myself what to think but it still doesn't stop me from wanting Adam to be whole, fit and happy.

After Clinic we exercise our independence by ordering bathroom equipment in Wild Sage instead of the creamy colour George told us to order; Adam very, very pleased.

We spend a quiet afternoon and evening together; Pauline phones to say we can use her Milford house next week.

Wednesday 1 August
Adam bright; sees to the animals for me and goes off with Lennie so I slip over to hold Grandad's hand. He's unable to sit up in bed by himself, confused, worried, tears . . . I do my best.

This afternoon Nick calls in. Give him a cup of tea and, when he asks how things are, hear myself saying, All right thank you. He is genuinely concerned. *How can I possibly say everything's all right?* I guess what I mean is that there's nothing even he could do to help. Tell him I feel I owe my sanity, such as it is, to him and Ted over these last few months, and thank him. This reminds me I haven't seen Ted for some time, so go over and bring him up to date when Nick goes. Ted seems to think I should detach myself from Adam mentally: I can't for the life of me see how.

19

Thursday 2 August
On waking I realise I can hear the milk float splashing up the lane – the earth smells glorious after the night's rain.

Adam feels lazy again. I can't force a good time, it's best to throw out a few suggestions and then just go along with his wishes. We don't have to go out on expeditions, we can have a lovely time here at home, wrapped up in each other. How could I detach?

Is there such a thing as a person? I think I'm different, depending upon who I'm with, who I'm bouncing off at the time. Maybe we only truly exist as colonies, like bees and ants, one individual being incomplete, if not quite incapable of independent survival. There is only one person in this world I have to be able to live with, and that is me, yet I don't really know who I am. Is this the sort of thought Ted had in mind when talking of detaching myself from Adam, I wonder?

Friday 3 August
Adam wakes bright, breezy, full of energy again. Lennie arrives before breakfast, it's gunfire, shouts of Pow! Pow! and laughter with the toast and marmalade. When Lennie disappears, Adam goes off with Peter.

Grandad won't keep himself covered and thinks I'm George today. Deflates when he realises I'm not; says George does not tell the truth and do I have enough kittens to soak and he's worried it costs £25 to buy a marrow, will I make sure I get everything I want. Tell him everything is under control, nothing to worry about, I'm fine and he has no need to concern himself about money; he cries. *Do* I help him?

George phones to say he'll arrive tomorrow afternoon, and have I heard any news about his father, by the way? – as though he didn't know I go in to visit the old man whenever I can. I just don't understand him.

Adam tired after this morning's sorties.

Saturday 4 August
Lovely long letter from Vicki, who is having a great time with Justin's people in Australia. No mention of study courses, I note.

George comes with us to look at kitchen cabinets and things, arranges for a rep. to call in two weeks. Adam is interested and seems just as keen to have the kitchen smartened up as he is about his bathroom.

Sunday 5 August
This morning George, Adam and I go for a walk through the fields – the first time all together since Sheba. We collect water weed from the river to bring back to the fish. George overtired, makes absolutely outrageous remarks I try to ignore, seems to want to pick a fight but there's no fight in me. Complains his house-hunting activities haven't got any further, but as he's spent the week between Brussels and Antwerp how could they, and no wonder he's tired. Seems to want to score off me all the time, which is irritating. Not a successful weekend.

Monday 6 August
Willow and Chris will see to the animals for us while we're away at Pauline's, and Adam is so excited while we see to the last-minute business of packing up and leaving the house. We stop for a leisurely lunch in a pretty pub garden, doodle on again with Adam feeding his favourite tapes into the car cassette player. We both enjoy the journey, her directions are superb and we arrive at Milford to a lovely welcome around 3:00. She shows us the house and immediate area, we have tea then she goes back to Gerrards Cross.

Adam and I go for a walk along the sea front – it's warm and sunny with a stiff breeze. Adam tells me when he's ready to turn round and go back. We relax a while, he's recharged his energy level so we walk along to explore the village, looking in shop windows and reading menus outside pubs and restaurants. Adam decides he's hungry. We go into a pub, he orders melon and half a roast duckling – not only does he finish that lot, he clears half my giant prawns too! Enjoys his meal tremendously, talks well, laughs and smiles, is altogether beautifully responsive and a joy to be with. We stroll back to the house, settle down for the night.

Tuesday 7 August
We sleep well, wake to find an overcast day. Set off for Bucklers' Hard, which is now commercialised beyond belief and £2.40 to park! We walk gently along the riverbank, there are plenty of things to watch. Go on a short boat trip, see all the boats and waterfowl. Visit some of the eighteenth-century cottages and the Maritime Museum. It starts raining in earnest, so we go to have lunch, hoping the weather will improve while we eat. Adam polishes off avocado with crabmeat, followed by scampi, and enjoys it so much he purrs! It pleases me so much when something really pleases him.

After lunch we drive around in the New Forest, stopping in various places to watch the ponies with their foals, walk by streams or just enjoy new places. Back at Milford Adam puts his feet up and watches television, I have a large mug of coffee.

Recharged, in our own ways, we set off again, this time exploring the coast to the west. Stop at Avonmouth Beach and walk along to the Quay at Mudeford – lots of families fishing for crabs, boats to watch, seagulls on one-legged sentry-duty on rocks – plenty for us to enjoy. We buy fresh prawns and a lobster to take home for supper and Adam purrs again as we eat our messy, sticky meal. Baths and early bed after our unaccustomed intake of sea air and all the walking we've done today.

Wednesday 8 August
We take a picnic to the beach at Friars Cliff but Adam is disappointed – beach shingly, totally unlike the expanse of white sands of my childhood, and the sea very cold. I'd warned him, but he isn't used to British coastal waters and it all comes rather as a shock. So, we come back and play cards on the patio. When the sun seems a little stronger, so does Adam and we walk down on to the shingle here. Adam bathes and enjoys it enough to want to swim again tomorrow. Steak and salad in front of the television, a stroll along the cliffs at dusk.

Thursday 9 August
Go to Keyhaven and take the ferry over to Hurst Castle. We enjoy the boat trip but don't think much of the castle. Lobster lunch on the way back, then onto the beach. He bathes again, we mark out a target area and play a stone-tossing game, make

friends with a dog. Bathe off sand and salt, go down to the village for supper – he has giant prawns and duckling. As we walk back, holding hands and swinging our arms, he says he's happy, so happy. Me, too.

Friday 10 August
A beautiful morning to wake up to. We bundle a few things into a bag and set off for Keyhaven, where I'm early enough to park free for once – glee! We watch the boats and swans in the sunshine, then get onto our ferry for the Isle of Wight. The moment she moves off at 9:45 – the bar opens! How could they. We watch sea birds on the mud flats, other boats, the spray flies and Adam loves it.

We decide to go on a coach tour of the island – my cosseted offspring is more used to cars than coaches – and stop in Ryde for lunch, after which we watch two men on water scooters like the ones we've seen in a James Bond film. One is expert, the other has to swim with his ashore after capsizing. Back at Yarmouth we watch the boats around the harbour – Adam is fascinated to see quite small children zipping around in inflatable dinghies with flip-up outboard motors, showing great expertise in their handling. And we notice that almost every boat has a dog on board.

Back home he's too interested in television to want to go out for supper. I make scrambled eggs with ham sliced up into it, with a side salad. This is not up to the standard to which he is rapidly becoming accustomed, and he announces firmly that we'll eat supper out tomorrow!

Saturday 11 August
Not such an easy day. Adam engrossed in Saturday-morning television so I go shopping in the village, buy steak for Sunday, a bottle of champagne to leave in the fridge as a thank you for Pauline and John.

Adam doesn't want to go off anywhere, complains of tummy ache. We play cards for hours, sitting out on the patio. He nibbles a ham sandwich for lunch, has six or seven petit mal turns, the first for ages. Brightens up later, is in a good mood again as we walk along the beach, decides he wants to go out for supper – he chooses duckling yet again so his tummy must be feeling better.

Sunday 12 August
He wakes very early, bright-eyed and bushy-tailed. We set off to visit a Butterfly Farm about three miles the Southampton side of Lyndhurst. They have tropical butterflies as well as British ones – huge gaudy floppy things bumbling about amid the tropical plants. Beautiful plants and pools. So many butterflies you have to be careful where you step, and one sat on my head which makes Adam laugh. Some of them have fantastic pupa cases. There are outside dragonfly pools with fish in them too – lots of creatures to watch. We go on a wagon ride through the forest; pleasant, but the horse is small and tired-looking, not a patch on Chris' shire horses. A simple but very good lunch there, then we move on to visit a dairy farm.

While I stroke one small calf, another creeps up behind me and starts sucking my elbow, a peculiar sensation which makes me jump – Adam of course thinks it hilarious! Ducks, hens, goats, sheep, pigs, pheasants, turkeys – Adam's favourites are the rabbits. He spends over an hour sitting in the large straw-filled pen, sometimes stroking them but mostly just watching the baby rabbits playing together. Do I owe him a large rabbit pen?

We watch the milking in a fully-computerised herringbone milking parlour – even the cows seem to know a lot, seem far from bucolic! All this is run by two men and a student and it's most impressive.

We're both very thirsty when we get back, have several long cold drinks but it doesn't revitalise Adam, who merely wants to play cards all evening.

When I'm reviewing the day as I tuck him into bed, a slip of the tongue has me referring to a dairy herd of butterflies – he laughs until he cries! It's a pretty idea, isn't it.

Monday 13 August
Up early to clean and tidy, pack up. We can't find anywhere nice to stop for lunch, just an ordinary grotty chain-type place, but for once Adam overcomes his scruples and eats self-service.

When we arrive home we find Vic's van in the drive and all sorts of rubbish on the lawn. Adam immediately falls to and helps demolish and dispose of the spare room wall, while Vic disconnects old bathroom fixtures.

We find 11 bantam babies; Adam thrilled, Mother Bantam

fierce. She can't possibly remember that we gave away the last ones? Later, the senior bantams won't go to bed and Adam gets furious with them. Then we understand: we see Mother Bantam chasing them off. Christen her Attila the Hen.

Tuesday 14 August

Clinic. It's vincristine day, so Outpatients at 9:00, where Dr Keith tells us he was staying with his parents in Barton at the same time we were in Milford, the next village along the coast. Adam and I decide that it was being brought up within sight of the Needles which influenced his choice of career. He manages his needle well this morning; Adam hangs onto my hand, holds his breath and it all happens easily amid repartee from Maxine, Dr Keith and me. Maxine suggests Dr Keith's wife bring their baby to Clinic to show us one day. I say, Yes, do ask her – a paediatrician having a baby is a declaration of faith. Why do I remember all this so clearly?

Up to Level 3 for coffee with some of the others while we wait for the blood test results, catching up with the news and laughing a lot. Dominic is in for platelets, Louise came in to be 'topped up' before they went on holiday, to make sure she was fit. I say, We've been very lucky, Adam hasn't had to go back in to the Ward since February; everyone says how well he looks, and he's growing, too.

Downstairs, Maxine asks Adam to stay in the waiting area, calls me in first. Dr Morrison says he's sorry to say that Adam's disease has come back. Everything goes black but I don't quite faint. He says that they'll do a bone-marrow to confirm it, but with 30% of his white cells being blasts, there's no doubt. As we've decided against transplantation – in his opinion, rightly – our options are either to have him in and give him massive chemotherapy again, which would make him feel rotten but may give him another four months after which he would relapse once more; or we could let this take its course, in which case they would give him platelets to stop any bleeding and plenty of analgesics so he wouldn't hurt or be frightened. I ask why another bone marrow if they are so sure; he agrees another routine blood test next week should confirm, a bone marrow isn't essential. I ask if Adam would have to come into the Ward, or could I keep him at home. Dr Morrison says if our family doctor is helpful I could manage at home; that he thinks sometimes in the past not enough morphine has been given, but he'd talk to our doctor about appropriate dosage; that there would always be a bed for Adam on 4B, where he knows the staff, should I wish him to come in at any time. Tell him Nick is extremely helpful, has made a point of involving himself, I'm sure he'd do anything he could; and as long as I could manage, keep him comfortable, I feel home is the right place for Adam to be. Dr Morrison holds my hands for a moment, says he's so sorry and that he doesn't like to think of me sitting alone in the house with my dying child. Say I think it may be easier like that. He says he'd like to talk to George and me together tomorrow, would 12:30 be all right. I agree.

Maxine takes me into the next room, makes me coffee, tells me I would not be alone anyway, that's what she's for, to phone her any time I want to. Asks if I'm sure we can get in tomorrow without Adam's knowing where we are going – reply that I'll fix it somehow. Stop shaking quite so much, go back in to Dr Morrison, Maxine brings in Adam and they exchange a few words, Dr Morrison writes up full treatment and says, Back next week.

Maxine joins us while we wait at pharmacy, makes Adam smile a few times, asks after Victoria, says she'll visit us soon. I thank her, tell her we're all right. Drive home very, very carefully, aware that I shouldn't be on the road.

Adam dives off to watch television so I go over to Ted. It's just an hour since they told me. Ted holds my hands and says, Come in – whatever's the matter? Tell him and he hugs me – exactly what I needed. He agrees Nick would do all he could to help me care for Adam at home, that that is the right thing to do. Tell him I've a problem about what to do with Adam tomorrow so he won't know where we are going. He promptly comes round with me and invites Adam to help him work in his orchard tomorrow with the baby tractor, and to have lunch with him. Adam is delighted, he likes Ted and Briony very much.

Go upstairs and make a discreet phone call to George, tell him about tomorrow's appointment and why; say if he can come down tonight he can tell Adam he's here to visit Grandad on his birthday, so his appearance in the middle of the week will be justified. He's dreadfully upset and says he has problems his end but that he'll be down tonight, somehow. It's still morning, yet today has already been an eternity.

Toasted cheese sandwiches and salad for lunch then Adam comes into Thame with me. He isn't much interested in food shopping, but helps me choose two boxes of chocolates for Grandad, select and write birthday cards, and we take them in to him. He's hardly coherent when he wakes, tries to eat a birthday card which Adam gently removes, substituting a chocolate. We don't stay long. It isn't necessary; he's hardly in this world now.

The electricity is off when we get home – feel like screaming. Laugh instead, get out the picnic stove and calor gas, light oil lamps and candles; George, Adam and I manage somehow to have an enjoyable supper. What is reality, after all?

When Adam is asleep I explain our options to George and tell him I feel strongly that we should not opt for further intensive chemotherapy but do our best to keep him happy and comfortable now. I don't feel I could put my Adam through all that chemotherapy again, knowing how bad he would feel, probably worse than last time, for the sake of a few more winter weeks. George says he isn't as strong as me, he couldn't make a decision which would mean Adam would die. I say he's probably going to do that fairly soon anyway: let's help him do it in the nicest possible way. A short life is not necessarily an incomplete one.

My mind is absolutely blown, like the electricity. How can I be so positive?

20

Wednesday 15 August
Adam excited at the prospect of going over with the tractor to help Ted. I suddenly remember the kitchen planner is due here at any minute, it's too late to stop him. It seems absolutely ludicrous, incongruous in the extreme, to be trying to talk about kitchens, but George is probably right when he says it's as good a way as any to spend the morning. It gives us something to hold on to, and probably keeps us sane. I doubt sanity entered the rep.'s opinion of us.

Watch Adam chug over the lane on the baby tractor, George and I set off for the JR. I feel wobbly, George allows me the concession of a cigarette in the car. Why am I wobbly, I've already heard it?

Dr Morrison is so kind and gentle, very much against reconsidering transplantation, even against putting Adam through more intensive chemotherapy; says the maximum time that could buy would be half the length of his first remission, i.e. four months, one of which would be spent in hospital feeling absolutely rotten. Explains in his opinion it'd be better to keep Adam happy now. I wonder slightly hysterically if he can thought-read me, or if this is really what he thinks. I don't realise until afterwards that our conversation yesterday told him the way my mind was working.

He explains they'd give antibiotics to alleviate any distressing infection, platelets to stop haemorrhage which is upsetting, continue to give normal maintenance treatment and Clinic visits which might buy a little useful time and would maintain contact and normality of routine. If he thought it appropriate he would cut down or cut out some of the treatment programme. Praises the effects of morphia which he says is a very useful drug. Promises to write to Nick, asks if there is anyone else I'd like him to write to, asks about friends and neighbours, is pleased when I tell him I have some super neighbours and live opposite Ted and Briony. He offers to write to them but

I tell him they already know, Adam is with Ted now. Assure him Nick is both helpful and sympathetic. A horrendous conversation – I do hope he doesn't have to do that sort of thing too often, poor man. But he does it so well, and managed to edge George off the transplantation line beautifully.

Geore is due to take Adam off on the longboat soon and is understandably getting cold feet about it. He says that Adam should be within 10 miles of the JR at all times.

Thursday 16 August
Vic and Chris appear early to take out the old bath. Chris wants it as a drinking trough for his horses so they need it out in one piece, quite an undertaking with a 6 foot cast-iron bath, narrow stairs. Adam watches, and when they go we play cards. He doesn't want his lunch, just jelly, then another few hours' cards. We both have our hair cut at Viv's, he has his done really short. Then he goes off in the Land Rover with Chris and Willow to see about some timber while I visit my psychotherapist.

It's not so easy this time. I say, How can I learn to help my Adam to die with dignity, and he says, Perhaps you should rather help him to live his life to the full first, so as not to prolong the dying part for either of you. Point taken, I think I already have that firmly in mind, but it is inevitably the unknown part which is the most troubling. No one can tell me how it's likely to happen. Without dwelling on it too much, I just can't make it go away, out of my mind. My mind goes a complete blank, I feel I'm wasting my time with him. He stays calm and receptive, says silence is okay, but it doesn't *feel* okay.

Chris and Adam are pumping out the pool when I get back, then he goes off on his bike with Lennie. He returns dreadfully upset because he's lost his precious bunch of keys – he thinks while he and Lennie were out. We retrace steps and spend a couple of hours searching, give up as the light fails. No good. Calm him down, cook him a second supper, help him bath – and when he climbs into bed we discover the keys – under his duvet. He's so pleased, and it's a great relief to me.

Friday 17 August
We set off early to the Cotswold Wildlife Park, armed with picnic. See just about everything; I think the two favourites this time are the meerkats and the ring-tailed coatis, which have lots of delightful playful babies. Adam does a lovely imitation of the rather supercilious meerkats; we think they look like senior members of the Board of Directors.

We ride on the miniature train, we admire all the owls, shudder at the crocodile, laugh at the antics of the monkeys, discuss the possibility of adopting a spider for Vicki who is terrified of them; we have a great time but our appreciation of wildlife does not extend to the wasps which want to join in the picnic.

George comes home, says not a lot until Adam's in bed, then is full of sarcastic remarks to me like, he'd have thought I'd want to spend every available moment with my child but, never mind, he could no doubt manage Adam on the boat. I reminded him that when he first told me about this proposed trip I asked whether he wanted me to come too and he said no, so I'd gone ahead and made other appointments. He just snaps, All right, don't make a big production out of it. I do not understand him at all. He can take Adam away for a few days and I'm damned if he's going to make me feel guilty about allowing it. I can use the time to begin to arm myself for what is to come by having time to talk freely to Nick, see Duncan, etc.

Saturday 18 August
A warm sunny day so all three of us set off to Thorpe Park, a pale imitation of Disneyland but interesting enough. We go on the ferry to the farm and wander around there, take a land train to Treasure Island, where the train is held up by pirates – very exciting and rather wet! Walk back to the restaurant, have a very good lunch, then we stroll round again, play a wild game of crazy putting, go on the Magic Mill boat trip which is pleasantly cool on such a baking day. When Adam is tired we come across an artist doing pastel portraits. He's so tired he sits still for her, and it's most interesting to watch the portrait develop – it goes through a stage of showing Adam as I imagine he would look at fifty, then comes back to being him right now, 14 and tired and ill. She saw that, too.

Sunday 19 August

Start the day by taking fresh flowers to Granny's grave and tidying around, which has been on my conscience for a few days, although with the temperature in the 80s flowers don't last long. Even so, why me and not George, when he's here. She's his mother, after all. I'm the one who feels that if you have a grave at all it should be nicely kept; I guess that's why me.

George has chairs out in the garden. He's planning a boating holiday for us all in Scotland next month. It's too hot for Adam in the sun, we sit on the rug in the shade of the plum tree and play cards. George barbecues lunch, Adam eats well, it's all fun and we play cards again. I almost beg for Shut-the-Box, Safari Round-up, Snakes and Ladders, *anything*, but no, it has to be cards.

George goes to see his father on his way back to London after lunch; maybe that's why he gets short and cross before he goes. He'll be back early on Wednesday for Adam.

Monday 20 August

Leave Adam helping Chris and Peter while I shop.

Tuesday 21 August

Full Clinic. Dr Keith officiates, says Adam is fine, platelets and haemoglobin okay, white cell count low but no funny cells, he's in remission again. No treatment for the next two weeks to let his white count come back up again, and they can give him his vincristine just before we go away next time, no problem.

I feel as weak, tearful, sick and shaky as I did after last week's Clinic. I think I can see what has happened: they gave him so much chemotherapy last week that, okay, it's knocked out the blasts, but he can't tolerate that level of treatment which also knocks his white cell count so low he'll have absolutely no immune system, which is why they've stopped treatment for two weeks now. Anyway, the words used were Remission Again – maybe one should sometimes deny imagination and live as though there's no tomorrow.

On our return I phone the office and leave a two-word message for George: Remission Again. He phones me back mid-afternoon, all excited and asking me to reassure him there wasn't a mistake, either last week or this week. He sounds ecstatic, and I'd thought him more of a realist than me. Then he tells me shyly that he had dinner last night with a priest who has no small reputation as a faith healer, and who promised to say some special prayers for Adam. Now this happens – a miracle, says George. I find I can't mention my theory – it *is* only my theory, I know nothing about the subject really. But it is indeed a miracle if it has given George the confidence to take his son off on the boat happily. I'm sure this trip will be of great value to them both. Dammit, I feel like George's mother as well as Adam's.

He also tells me he thinks he's found a house, it'll need a lot spending on it and it isn't what he wants but he can't afford what he wants, it'll have to do.

Mr Burrett appears on crutches this morning to help in the garden. I know, both he and his wife have told me, his doctor says he should keep on working, but good heavens! I feel like Hitler.

Adam enjoys a good supper, does most of his packing before early bath and bed.

Wednesday 22 August
Adam up early putting the finishing touches to his packing, seeing to the chicks and ducks for me, feeding Cat. We put recharged batteries into his torch, then he has nothing to do, so ... we play cards. George arrives 10:30, much sighing, clutching of head, George has been busy, George is tired. Have I bought them supplies, he asks. No, I say, you told me when I asked that you'd do that on your way up, remember. Oh, I'm far too tired to go shopping, he says, so Adam and I go down to the little shop while George gives himself a shot in the arm by making a few phone calls. When he's finished phoning he decides they should eat something here before they leave for the boat. Do sausages, bacon, egg and tomatoes on toast for them, and at last they're off. Vic and Chris hammer away upstairs.

Duncan arrives for lunch with me and I explain to him the events of the last two Tuesdays. Sadly, he confirms my suspicion that full treatment shot everything down temporarily; in other words we're between the devil and the deep blue sea.

Adam can't tolerate full treatment and only full treatment could keep this at bay a little longer.

Duncan doubts whether we have as long as two or three months. Says he wouldn't be inclined to give platelets, because bleeding and not replacing the blood helps them to die of anaemia, a nice way to die. He agrees that here at home is the best place for Adam to be, and thinks I could manage it. He says we should tell Vicki what the situation is, and that I should go to my mother when Adam dies. I tell him one can go to classes to prepare oneself for childbirth; this is I think far more important yet I feel totally unprepared to help Adam to have a good death. He says, Yes, you need a nice midwife to help Adam be reborn gently.

I feel so lucky to know him – he talks about all these things so naturally, in such a domestic setting, it all becomes much more real to me.

I can feel Adam, not here, not in his room at the end of the house. This is, as Duncan pointed out, a trial run at life without him. Go to bed but don't sleep. This is dreadful.

Thursday 23 August

Remove two dead mice – contributions from Cat – from the front doorway, one dead hedgehog from the pond; can't get away from death. Thought: death is the only certainty in life.

Go see Nick. Dr Morrison's letter arrived yesterday, he says, he was planning to call on me today, but I beat him to it. He tells me that he personally will be available at any time, day or night, unless he's away in which case he'll make sure I have someone else who's been primed by him to call on. He wonders again whether Helen House could help. I explain I want Adam at home if possible, and if he has to be anywhere else, 4B at the JR, where he knows the staff and they know him. I don't feel it appropriate to involve another set of people at this stage. He says Helen House people help to keep dying children at home, it isn't simply a place for them to die in, as I had thought.

Tell him Maxine is coming to lunch tomorrow, ask if he would like to come too and meet her if he's free. He sounds enthusiastic; he really wants to be part of the team and liaise with the hospital people to help Adam all he can. He's super. Aren't I lucky in these doctors I know: Duncan, Ted and Nick.

Friday 24 August
Make watercress soup and various cold dishes for lunch. Mrs Burrett calls in the middle with grandchild to collect feathers and some early apples – she kindly makes up for the interruption by hanging out my washing for me!

Maxine arrives first, Nick soon after. They're both so very nice they feel more like family than guests – they're 'kitchen' people, they fetch and carry and make themselves at home. I guess that's why they are both so good at their jobs: they can relate easily. They have a friend in common and talk easily from the start.

I won't need anyone from Helen House or elsewhere: Maxine says she'll be here as often as I want her, and if it means staying three or four nights at the end, that is what she will do. She and Nick swap phone numbers and she says she'll keep in touch with him about the blood counts. They both seem delighted to have had the opportunity to meet and I'm glad they appear to get on so well. Nick promises to drop in frequently and says he'll come to lunch with Adam and me next Friday.

Maxine stays on a while, says they wouldn't let Adam suffer or bleed from the nose and throat for six weeks like the boy in the *Reader's Digest* article someone kindly gave me – she says they would give platelets and send him home again. She stresses how much Dr Morrison cares about the children in his care; says he sometimes gives parents the impression he's abrupt, but that's because he cares so much. That is exactly the impression I have of him – that he cares deeply for the children above all. She can't tell me how it's likely to happen, either; bleeding, an infection, failure of some important organ.

Feel rather light-headed when she leaves. Here am I, trying to set up handy arrangements for the death of my child, my Adam. It's a sensible thing to do, but so unreal it's mind-bending.

Saturday 25 August
I wish I had more faith. My prayers for my children have always been on the lines of, Please God take care of them, give them the strength to do this or that to the best of their ability, rather than asking for specifics for them such as to win this or pass that. I have asked God to help me find some place where

Adam will be able to lead a happy, secure and fulfilling life after my death: why don't I have the conviction that He is doing just that, albeit in an unexpected way, and feel able to accept it.

Take some roses up to Granny's grave, tidy round. The Church is locked so I can't go inside. Pray a formless prayer, with much passion, in the Churchyard, which is beautiful and so serene.

At home I drink more coffee and just sit, for about an hour.

Go see Grandad, who wakes, just about, as I go in; knows me and is pleased to see me, goes back to sleep. He reawakens with hiccoughs. I make some bright remark about his having spent the night on the tiles, obviously, and he says, Oh yes please, Katherine, I'd like that, Katherine, and he's asleep again. After another ten minutes or so of holding his hand, I shake him gently and say I'll come back when he's feeling more awake. The inside of his mouth looks ulcerous and there's a covered tray in his room marked Mr Adair, Mouth Tray.

See Sister on my way down, she says he's gradually going. Explain why I won't be able to visit so frequently now and she says in his present condition he won't notice, not to worry, I've been in often when it mattered, and am I all right, she doesn't know what to say. I'm all right but I don't know what to say, either.

Do some gardening, there's a good deal of comfort in a garden. It's a living thing which responds not only to hard work, satisfying in itself, repetitive, rewarding, but also to love and creativity. Although, looking at my garden now, you'd never believe it could mean a lot to me; poor thing has been sadly neglected. I gain a sense of composure, gradually. Plants die or die back but there is still life there, in the root or in seeds scattered in the soil to grow up in another season; there is always promise, hope, even in the blackest time of the year. When I pull out the dead sweet peas I don't cry because they are over, I smile to recall how pretty they were, how profuse, how sweet-smelling. Life goes on; even though things die, in a way they go on for ever and there's an interdependence as well as a battle for survival. Sometimes things almost make sense, then it slips away again.

It's mighty lonely around here.

Sunday 26 August
Briony calls round. Yes, she would like some of the asparagus plants in a couple of weeks, and she is one hundred percent behind the decisions we have made on Adam's behalf; that is just the way she would have chosen if it had been a child of hers. That's a lovely thing to know. She says she went daily to give an injection to someone who had relapsed and that she didn't think people should have to go through all that for nothing, those last few months seemed terrible. Says she knows how hard this is for George and me in our different ways, but is quite sure we are doing the right thing, and isn't it nice for me that Vicki is happily occupied elsewhere so I can concentrate on Adam. Yes indeed. She's super and I'm so grateful to her and Ted for their assurances.

Garden and think. And sit without thinking.

Very slowly burn some fish for supper. Don't eat it. Neither does Cat.

Monday 27 August
Garden again, come in and look at a pan of soup for a while at lunchtime then throw it away as Cat isn't any more interested in it than I am. Walk down to the Church. It's locked again. I feel shut out, excluded, don't know why I feel so upset about it, my God doesn't live in Church, that's only His office. Spend some time sitting in the Churchyard, a lovely place to be. Rooks noisy in the trees; a Siamese cat striding determinedly with head held high but his rabbit is so large it still trails along the ground.

Gardening again, I think if I could only invent a gourmet recipe for bindweed and ground elder, they'd instantly disappear from the garden. It's very hot.

George phones – they've had a good time, Adam fit, very helpful, good with the boat and enjoying things, eating like a horse, but they need baths so they're coming home tomorrow evening.

Tuesday 28 August
Visit Grandad. He's very dribbly, his eyes look sore, his skin so thin you feel he must have no substance at all. I stay another 15 minutes watching him sleep, then tell him I'm going now, have a nice sleep. Oh Katherine, is that what you think it is?

Oh Katherine. Leave, feeling sad, sick and for some reason slightly resentful.

Ted calls and hugs me, says soothing things and is such a comfort. It's beautiful, the way both he and Duncan hug me; it seems to recharge me so I can pass it on, to Adam and to Grandad.

Go and see my therapist. With Ted I felt relaxed enough but with him I'm very uptight, everything seems so extremely painful again. And it feels rather like prostitution, this: baring the most intimate part of oneself to a stranger, by appointment, for money. It just doesn't feel right. He talks about my taking on too many responsibilities, running up an emotional deficit. Maybe, but if you care for people you can't suddenly stop because you've decided you are already using up the amount of concern and prayer you feel free to offer. I don't feel it is something within my control. Adam obviously comes first by miles. In an odd way it may even be beneficial to Adam to have my anxieties slightly diffused: too much anxiety directed towards him may be a burden on him and detrimental – he can pick up my feelings and I try hard to project positive feelings towards him.

Realise with shame that I have put people I love into the background just now: Victoria and my mother. Not quite out of sight out of mind, but because there's nothing I can do for them, other than write letters, they are undoubtedly in the back of my mind.

George and Adam come back happy, both enjoy a hot bath.

When we've had supper and Adam is in bed, I tell George gently that it wasn't a miracle, it was a natural consequence of the medication. He argues. Don't press it, but thank him for Adam's boat trip and tell him how very useful these few days have been to me, giving me the opportunity to see Duncan, Nick, Maxine. He knows Duncan and has met Nick but doesn't know them as well as I do, hasn't met Maxine at all, and can't really understand.

Wednesday 29 August
Adam fine, George irritable in his disappointment and looking for something to be wrong. He's convinced the builders' merchants have sent me the wrong lavatory and bidet – why didn't I check and send them back. Quietly show him the catalogue

and he can't deny I got what I had ordered and he had approved. The lavatory seat isn't the same as the one in my bathroom – he unpacks it, raising steam, then decides he likes this one better. After a long discussion with Chris he decides that the bath needs to be moved two inches.

I must have washed his new Lacoste T-shirt with something coloured, he says, Look, you've ruined it, it cost more than £20. It's just rather grubby. He goes to visit his father, comes back to lunch after which he seems reluctant to leave although he has me so strung up I'm longing for him to go and trying hard not to show it. He cries. He won't let me touch him, but I tell him I think we're doing well for Adam at least, if not for us. He won't let me talk any more; he goes back to London.

Play endless games of cards with Adam and a little Snakes and Ladders; we laugh a lot. He has two new jokes: I couldn't sleep last night because of all the planes flying round my room. *Planes*, Adam, why were they flying round your room? Because I left the landing lights on! And, Which is the smartest, a parrot or a chicken? A parrot, of course – you never heard of Kentucky Fried Parrot, did you!

Thought: A gentle death must be the finest gift of life. And, as Duncan said, death must be good when it replaces pain, uncertainty; it's a very different thing if it happens by accident and replaces happiness and wellbeing.

Thursday 30 August
Adam a little sleepy, watches Vic and Chris work rather than come out with me. When I return within the hour he's dressed and playing with Lennie.

We go to lunch with Thea, who responds admirably to Adam's new jokes! Rowdy lunch; Adam admires Sam and the gentle Annabel while the two smallest girls amuse him no end. They all disappear to watch a video on television and Thea and I have a quiet talk. She thinks from her experience with her baby that I would manage better if George weren't underfoot while Adam is in extremis; he'd probably feel he ought to be there from a sense of duty, but wouldn't be able to take it and would cause me problems. My feelings exactly. I think he'd get too emotional and demanding at a time when I'd rather concentrate entirely on Adam. I wouldn't dream of denying George presence, but would rather not go out of my way to invite him.

When we weigh ourselves at bathtime we discover Adam has gained 7lb. and I've lost 7lb. this week!

Friday 31 August
Adam dozy again and doesn't want to play outside with Lennie. We play cards while Vic hammers away at pipes upstairs, then Adam watches television while I make lunch.

Nick tries very hard to talk to Adam, who just won't respond, doesn't seem to remember anything about his boat trip. Horace escapes from the orchard again after lunch, we chase him back and play again.

Later Adam perks up, goes off with Lennie and, great excitement, they see the fire engines putting out a fire in the store-room of the little shop.

Saturday 1 September
George here in time for lunch, after which we smarten up and go into London. First we go look at George's new house, a three-bed, two-bath Victorian terrace with a small garden in a very nice area near the river. It was rented out so isn't in good decorative order but George will do it up nicely, he's good at that. There's an impressive five-foot sunken circular bath in the main bedroom/dressing room/bathroom suite, for orgies or rugby teams rather than the solitary pursuit of cleanliness . . . Me, I can't get used to London houses, so tall and narrow it invariably makes me feel I'm living on a staircase and I keep forgetting which floor I'm on. Still, it isn't for me to live in. Wonder if he could sink his sunken bath into the garden, plug up the plug-hole and keep goldfish in it.

We meet some friends of George with their children at Drury Lane Theatre and all enjoy seeing '42nd Street', a lovely dinner afterwards at an Italian restaurant. One of the other children fades, but not Adam – he's really enjoying himself.

Sunday 2 September
I go to early service. George goes to see his father, finds the old man asleep so comes straight home again.

Angela and Alan come for lunch. We all love them and it's a great success. George is just about to leave for London when

Matron phones to tell him his father is ill and they've sent for the doctor. She rings after examining Grandad and George is left with the impression that his father will die of pneumonia within the next 48 hours or so. He sets off to visit him, intending to go straight on to London, but changes his mind and comes back here so he can visit again in the morning before going to work.

Monday 3 September
My solicitor says I should get what sounds to me to be a fantastic maintenance payment, far more than I need. I explain the family situation, say I don't need all that anyway, I would like George to propose an allowance rather than ask for one, and ask him to get in touch with George with a view to their meeting. I must be a disappointment to him!

Take Adam to have lunch at Thea's once again, while I go on to the Gilbert's. Ruth has some friends there, we all have drinks and a lovely lunch around the pool. I hadn't realised before how much death comes into general conversation. Ruth and her group go off, Duncan and I disappear into his study.

He asks me a lot of questions about how Adam seems, about Grandad, about how I'd felt alone in the house when Adam and George were on the boat – tells me that was good practice for me, and how terrible I am going to feel when Adam dies; how he and Ruth and their friends do talk about death, at their ages they have to face it and speaking of it helps it become a reality, not just something which happens to other people. He talks of relationships, parent and child as well as husband and wife; of illness and death and loneliness and leukaemia and attitudes to these things. I have a strong feeling I still have a lot to learn from this man, and he's so natural in the manner in which he speaks of the unspeakable I think I do absorb a lot, accept a lot. I wonder if he has any idea how much he is helping me, how many dragons he slays for me. He says he's sorry *he* can't become my lover and cuddle me better; when I say, Oh no, he says, Well, someone should. I think he is loving me far more intimately by helping me through this extremely painful time like this than if we had gone to bed together, which wouldn't seem right.

Collect Adam from Thea's and stop off to see Grandad on the way back; Adam waits in the car playing tapes. Grandad doesn't seem any worse to me than he was last week; says Oh Katherine a few times, holds my hand and sleeps. Tell George this when he phones for news and he seems surprised. He comes back here at about 11:30 p.m., phones the nursing home to ask if he should go in tonight; they say No, thank you, so he goes to bed.

Tuesday 4 September
Adam happy helping Chris and Peter – he does so enjoy their working here, and they are super with him. I go off to buy some tiles for his bathroom. George sets off for the nursing home and phones later from London to say his father has rallied and the doctor says we're to go ahead with our plans for the Scottish holiday regardless – we're to go and not to telephone. George has spent the last couple of weeks surrounded by brochures and has planned a week swanning around Loch Ness in a boat. We should leave here on Thursday. When I see him after lunch the old man is deeply asleep, barely flickers an eyelid when I speak to him, touch him.

Adam spends another happy afternoon with Lennie and bicycles. He doesn't want supper, however, says his arms, legs and head hurt; he has a slight temperature but won't take any paracetamol.

Peter brought him a beautiful Roland Rat this afternoon; he goes to bed early cuddling it.

Wednesday 5 September
Adam and I leave for the JR at 8:30 calling gaily to Peter, See you in a couple of hours. Dr Keith takes blood sample – an extra large one – and gives Adam his vincristine.

We see Betty and Frankie – Dominic has been on the Ward for most of the last five weeks, with breathing problems, racing heart and temperature, not eating because his stomach hurts, only comfortable with his oxygen mask on.

The blood results take a long time but at last Dr Keith comes to look Adam over. Starts by peering into his eyes; says he wants a second opinion. We take Adam into the playroom, leave him with Carol for a moment while I follow Keith. He explains the blasts are back – 45% this time, although the rate of increase isn't so far significant, and that what he thinks he can see in the back of the retina indicates increased pressure inside Adam's head. He wants another doctor to have a look, see whether he can see it too. Other doctor does see the same thing; we're to stay and see Dr Morrison who will come before lunchtime. More coffee while we wait.

Dr Morrison sees the same as the first two doctors, explains it's an accumulation of leukaemic cells impeding bloodflow and causing pressure, which would lead to severe headaches, nausea and vomiting unless relieved. I ask if it's relieved with a lumbar puncture or drugs. He says primarily a lumbar puncture, but at the same time they'll put some methotrexate into the spinal column which, although it won't make any difference to the progress of the disease in the long run, will dissipate the leukaemic cells in there now.

He crosses the Ward to remove a ham roll half-way to Adam's mouth and explains to him that he'll be in overnight, they'll give him an anaesthetic about tea time and do the lumbar puncture to stop him getting headaches and we'll see how he feels tomorrow. Adam seems quite happy about that.

I come home to fetch him a few things, phone and leave a message with George's secretary to the effect that Adam and I will not be going to Scotland in the morning. Back in to keep Adam company, read to him – he seems to become progressively sleepier as the day goes on. We go down about 5:30, I stay with him as usual while he goes under, holding his hand, talking to him, stroking him. They do a bone marrow, too.

A coffee with Betty and Frankie, then back down with the nurse and Roland Rat to fetch Adam from the Recovery Room. He's quite with-it, only a little sleepy; soon has first one, then another glass of water and by 7:30 he's tucking into sausages and chips, telling me to go home.

George arrives shortly after me, is terribly jumpy and snappy, saying all the doctors he's ever had dealings with have been able to tell him the chances of something happening, when it'd happen, why can't these doctors? I think they have; they certainly don't withhold information but they aren't prophets and can't know exactly. He won't hear of our *not* going to Scotland. Try very hard to calm him down and explain Adam agrees it'd be much nicer to go on a boat on Loch Ness when he's feeling good and can enjoy it rather than when he may have blinding headaches and be sick. And how on earth can George, who a few weeks ago when the child seemed fit announced I shouldn't take him more than 10 miles from the JR, now, when things are looking dodgy, think I could contemplate isolating him on a boat in the middle of Loch Ness? A super holiday for him if all is well, sure, but in the circumstances out of the question. Poor George has put so much into planning this holiday, he can't see my point of view. I don't know, maybe I *am* irrational. I'm certainly led by my instincts.

Thursday 6 September
I set off for the JR, George stays here to ring the boatyards about the possibility of picking up a boat on Monday instead of Saturday, even though I've talked myself blue in the face about not going at all. It's so far away: home and the proximity of the JR spell security. I suppose he's at least keeping our options open.

Adam is dressed and feeling fine. Keith tells me no mercaptopurine because his platelets are low; the vincristine and prednisone should be sufficient just now to keep the white cells in order. Dr Morrison says I can take Adam home now and adds he doesn't think it'd be a good idea to take him off to Scotland – I almost kiss him, wonder again whether he's a mind-reader.

While Adam is at home with George, I slip into Aylesbury to see his head teacher, explain he won't be back at school, frankly there are more important things to do with the time. She's sweet, says if there's anything they can do for Adam or for me just let them know and they'll be very happy to do it.

George goes off to his meetings in Scotland; Adam helps Chris and Peter, then we spend the evening cuddling, watching television together.

Friday 7 September
While Adam watches Chris tile his bathroom I nip up to see the Vicar. Explain Adam knows nothing of it, but he has relapsed and probably only has a month or so now; I'd like him to bless Adam for me without his suspecting there's something funny going on. He suggests bringing Adam to a 10:30 communion, explaining he's not yet old enough to take the bread and wine, but bringing him to the altar rail with us to be blessed. And try to believe that, although we don't know

enough to be able to understand it now, what is happening may well be the best for Adam, hard as it is for those of us who love him.

I wonder if I really believe in God. Somehow the world is so intricately well-organised one can't doubt a divine creation – it seems impossible it all happened by accident. Yet sometimes I wonder if God exists simply because we need someone to be all-caring, all-forgiving, sometimes vengeful – we need also to think people like Hitler, Idi Amin, Col. Gadaffi and all the petty little Hitlers get their come-uppance some time, somewhere; we need to feel some divine being is there, holding up a notice saying The Buck Stops Here.

As to eternal life, I'm equally ambivalent: is it just that we are so egocentric we can't contemplate our own mortality? Yet the evolutionary development of the body seems so obvious to me that the long-term development and refinement of our souls, the more important part of us, also makes sense. Some people seem to be born older and wiser than others. And haven't we all met people we feel instantly in tune with, feel we've met before? What about infant prodigies, the geniuses? What is intuition if not a creative use of instinct, which is long-term memory, built in to us?

Adam, in fine form, wins numerous card games but has little appetite. Discovers little red spots on his feet at bedtime; puzzled but not disturbed. He'd seen them before.

Briony and Ted, God bless them, will be my safety line while Nick is away. If I ring the JR with a question, the junior doctors, for their own protection, would have to say, Bring him in: it's so reassuring to know there is someone I can sound out first, so I won't have to take him in unless it really is necessary. Nick even arranged an introduction to another nurse too, so I also have a Maxine substitute while she's away. (We all planned to be away at the same time.). They're all so kind and considerate.

Saturday 8 September

Adam spends a silent morning in pyjamas so I ask Ted if it's the petechiae (little red spots) indicating problems and should I do anything about them. He says no, they don't cause discomfort and won't get worse very quickly – the two things I wanted to know.

Hours and hours of board and card games. Playing with Adam is far more important than housework – it doesn't really matter that the carpet is wall-to-wall Lego, or that the kitchen floor crunches as we walk across it. The house is here for my convenience, after all, not I for its. Much better that Adam and I should feel free to relax into games or simply sitting and cuddling. Let the rest of the world go by.

George returns this afternoon. He's been to see if he could arrange an 'insiders' tour of Heathrow Airport, or organise anything else which might be of interest to Adam, who loves planes – bearing in mind that the last time we spent an afternoon on the Observation Deck there was a sudden waft of fumes from the aircraft, a girl fainted and Adam managed to be sick down the suit his father was wearing to a Board Meeting.

While I cook poppadoms and Adam comes through to 'test' them, George brings us all an excellent Indian take-away supper. Adam bright-eyed, looking a little fragile; we all laugh a lot and enjoy our evening.

Sunday 9 September
George takes Adam off with Chris, Willow and Peter to Wroughton in Wiltshire, a science museum open day – shire horses ploughing, traction engines working, exhibitions of planes, cars, etc. It's a cold day but they all have a good time and Adam and Peter have a helicopter ride! All return absolutely exhausted – except Adam, who is starving hungry but in better shape than any of them! I stay here, catch up on some housework, letter-writing. Although I keep busy, know he'll be back in a few hours, there's such a lost lonely feeling without him.

Monday 10 September
Another cold day and when Adam threatens to eat breakfast with his anorak on I look at the thermometer outside the kitchen window: 50° so I turn the heating on.

We're all short of inspiration about what to do with today, now we aren't going to Scotland. Eventually decide to go to Stratford. A pleasant drive, and we enjoy looking at some of the old houses, including one owned by Shakespeare's son-in-law, who was a doctor. Some of the medical implements on exhibition make us love Clinic – these tools seem more appropriate to Vic and plumbing than to people and hospitals. Whatever did he do with the fork in his medical kit? I think I'd rather not know!

Wonder if our little house is indeed as old as these.

We have a very good lunch in a hotel with appalling service, all eat well and laugh a lot. George teases me about which of us will pay for the improvements to my little house. I urge George to meet my solicitor, think it'd speed things up and that they'd get on. Oh, says George, Is he good, does he want a decent job? He says he will have to take my solicitor out to lunch, if it were the other way round he, George, wouldn't be able to stand the mark-up! Wants to know what maintenance he told me I should get; I won't tell him, say I'm far more interested in whatever figure George proposes himself.

We wander around Stratford again and see a coffer in an antique shop and because I almost guess what they were asking for it George buys it, sells it to Adam for 20p (all he has with him) and Adam gives it to me! Aren't men complicated. Luckily we came in my car, it fits in with the back seat folded down and I have a most uncomfortable journey home crouched down next to it in the back, arriving just before curvature of the spine set in permanently!

After supper George returns to London although he had previously arranged to have this week off for the Scottish trip. Adam goes up to his room, coughing. Give him hot lemon and honey, cough mixture, rub his chest with Vick. He settles nicely with Cat on one side of him and Roland Rat on the other.

I love that child so much it *must* protect him.

Tuesday 11 September
Clinic. Joanne takes the blood sample. Dominic is in Intensive Care, Betty and Frankie look terrible. Want to take them out to dinner, they both need a shot of something to revitalise them.

Drs Evelyn, Morrison and Keith all have a look in Adam's eyes. No active treatment.

Wednesday 12 September
While I'm stuffing laundry into the washing machine this morning it occurs to me that Betty and Frankie might have a

laundry problem while they're in the JR with Dominic. Adam and I go along to see them. Dominic is sitting up and looking interested in life, Betty looks a whole lot better. We have coffee on Level 3. She says laundry's under control at the moment and yes, they'd like to come out to dinner – will phone in the morning to confirm.

Adam and I go straight to Thea's for a late coffee, return the sleeping bag, sadly unused, borrowed for proposed boat trip, then go on to Karen's for lunch. She gives us fish and chips, a good bottle of wine and fruit pie and jelly. Adam eats masses, including nine-tenths of the fruit pie which pleases Karen. She and I have a lovely chat about trivialities. Most important, that, on occasion. Clever Karen.

During the evening Willow comes in, having temporarily mislaid Chris, but stays to have a drink with me. She says yes sure, she and Chris would be happy to watch television with Adam while George and I take Betty and Frankie out to supper tomorrow.

It's a lovely mild evening, Adam and I go for a walk around the fields after our supper – he strides out manfully while I trot behind trying to avoid thistles. It's great. Somehow our sensibilities are honed, we gain such tremendous enjoyment from such little things these days.

Thursday 13 September

Play cards, play cards, and then we play cards . . . Frankie rings at midday, says Dominic still brighter and back on 4B from Intensive Care, but they'll take a raincheck on dinner. He can't persuade Betty to leave him for that long, although he concedes it'd do them both good.

After lunch Adam goes off with Willow anyway to choose and watch videos. George back late – Justin's father unexpectedly called to see him. Victoria is settled well in Australia, she and Justin now living with other boys and girls in an apartment – or 'unit' as it is known in Australia – the Greens keeping a close eye on them. George has arranged trip to Heathrow tomorrow. Adam is extremely excited.

When he has his bath Adam notices a few more petechiae around his feet and legs. He has some brown freckles too; we decide he's looking very pretty and wonder whether he'll produce green or yellow polka dots as well. He's mildly interested, not at all bothered. It's so hard but I'm sure a calm casual approach is best.

Although he has a very soft toothbrush, his gums bleed a little when he does his teeth. He doesn't notice, I don't say anything.

Friday 14 September

Up at 6:30 as George and Adam want to leave early for the Airport in case there are hold-ups on the motorway. Adam leaves wreathed in smiles, looking very smart.

I slip up to the JR. Dominic looks much better and has his right arm free again. His eyes are huge and he's still not eating. He won't let Betty leave the room to have coffee with me.

Go straight on to see Grandad, who is asleep and a strange purple colour. Shake his shoulder gently, talk to him, but he doesn't wake. Breathing easy and steady. It doesn't seem fair to shake him again, so I just leave after a while. A nurse says he was like that yesterday too, and adds admiringly, He seems determined to hang on, doesn't he.

George brings Adam back about 4:30, Adam looking rather white and drained but they've had a super day. To Paris and back in TriStar, with Adam sitting behind and slightly above the Captain from pre-take-off to landing, both ways – he could see and hear everything that went on! The British Airways official in Paris met them and made a fuss of Adam when they arrived. They were given a lovely lunch and when they got back to Heathrow George's friend met them, showed them over Concorde which was being serviced *and* they wanted to move it so Adam sat in the Captain's seat of Concorde while it went up the runway from one hangar to another – he could pretend he was driving it, in control! That was all so thrilling for him, wonderful! He came home with a British Airways pen, a T-shirt, badge, Concorde pencil-sharpener, one very happy, sleepy boy. I wonder if these lovely people have any idea just how much pleasure they have given him – I'm bursting with gratitude.

Saturday 15 September

One of those days when the principal mistake seems to be waking up at all. Everything I say or do is wrong this morning; it takes supreme control not to scream at George. Why we can't give each other loving support in this situation instead of riling and draining each other I just do not understand.

Things do get better. No doubt we both make a tremendous effort. We all spend an enjoyable afternoon and evening together.

Sunday 16 September

George, Adam and I go to 10:30 communion. Adam between us at the altar rail, I hold the paten while the Vicar blesses him. I'm so pleased, somehow it means a lot to me.

We go round after the service to visit Granny's grave and George is furious with me because it was her birthday on the 14th and I forgot to get special florists' flowers. Why didn't I tell him I wasn't going to do that, he would have ordered something to be delivered. Tell George I'm sorry, I just forgot, it wasn't a positive decision not to do it; if I'd remembered I would have seen to it myself; I do have rather a lot on my mind at the moment and my memory was never my strong point. I'm so sorry this has upset him; please remember I care for her grave all the year round, do my best. He finds some roses and nicotiana in the garden, takes them to the Churchyard with maximum fuss. I feel whipped.

George wants lunch instantly, leaves for London straight after.

Adam, the root of my deepest distress, is also my greatest source of comfort.

22

Monday 17 September
Grey, thundery; Adam pale, quiet. Martha phones to tell me Dominic died. Poor Betty and Frankie, they all put up such a fight.

When I tell Adam, his comment is, lucky Dominic, he isn't hurting any more. Then he adds, But his poor Mummy and Daddy don't have a child now: maybe they'll have another baby to love. I feel very humble.

Tuesday 18 September
Clinic. No active treatment, back in two weeks.

Wednesday 19 September
Duncan comes in, saying he thinks I'm under a lot of strain just now and that the menopause can be a difficult time for some women, how old am I? – 45 – Oh, he says, You're all right, you've years yet! He's lovely, makes me laugh. He doesn't stay very long, but talks to me again about leukaemia, death, attitudes to dying, about marriage, about the difficulties of loving people. He's so sensible, such a caring sort of person, he brings a breath of fresh air to subjects which are usually hidden away. The experience of the mature combined with the enthusiasm and curiosity of the young: I think that is what makes him a very special person to know.

Thursday 20 September
A grey wet day but it's Thame Show and Adam is determined to go. We post our thank-you letters to George's friend and the British Airways' Captain, then set off to visit Grandad on our way to Thame. We can't wake him. Sister tells me the doctor found secondaries in his abdomen, that he has localised pain when he's moved, that they are controlling the pain with drugs. He'll take fluids if they remind him to swallow. Because he's so immobile he'll probably get pneumonia again. They

do keep moving him, to alleviate pressure problems too, but he prefers the foetal position. She thinks they have the pain under control.

The car park for the Thame Show is a horrific sea of mud – a policeman tells me to drive in and just keep driving; park with no problems.

We look at a fantastic variety of caged birds and rabbits – Adam's favourites – several craft exhibits, and there's a sudden downpour so we, like several hundreds of other people, head off looking for food and shelter. In one produce tent there's a sudden loud clap of thunder, we look up and see Mrs Wolf, Adam's teacher, for all the world as though she were produced by it, like a genie in a pantomime! Adam enjoys the encounter. We exchange a few light-hearted and dripping remarks, get some smoked salmon sandwiches for lunch.

We're both wet and uncomfortable so we decide to go home. The car drives easily out of the muddy field, thank goodness, as Adam begins to shiver. Hot baths immediately, change of clothes, light the heater in the sitting room, make hot drinks. Adam starts coughing again – I don't like the fumes from the heater, either. By bedtime he says he has a headache, but not enough of one to want anything for it. He promises to wake me if he wants anything in the night.

Friday 21 September
Adam quiet, no temperature but sniffing.

George phones to say he has to go shopping in the morning but will be back tomorrow afternoon. He's very rushed and hardly has time to listen to what I have to tell him about his father.

Saturday 22 September
Adam pale-faced, coughing in front of the television in his pyjamas all morning. Then we play cards . . .

This afternoon he walks down to Mandy's with me for eggs. George spots us and stops to give us a lift back home. He wants to talk about Victorian bathroom fittings for his London house.

He and Adam decide they want an Indian supper again and somehow, with the assistance of television, we do all have a happy afternoon and evening. I wish Jim could Fix-It for us.

Sunday 23 September
I had a night of nightmares. In one, I'd been accused of shoplifting and my father appears to say he'd like to help me but he isn't qualified. Then again, I've been to visit Grandad where I am suddenly bitten by the devil – a large purple bruise appears on my left arm with two round very deep holes which I can't quite see, so I phone Nick and Duncan to ask what I should do but neither know. Interesting.

Adam still coughing during the day but not badly, not at all at night.

Keep him company in the bathroom, give him cough mixture, hot lemon and honey, settle him down.

George is cross because molehills have appeared on the small area of grass immediately outside the front door. As though I'd issued an invitation.

Monday 24 September
George complains of a fox barking and keeping him awake. I slept very little but didn't hear it.

He sets off to see my lawyer. I expect him to phone during the evening to tell me about it, but he doesn't.

Adam and I spend a happy morning together then after lunch he goes to Willow's to watch more videos while I set off in the rain to Dominic's funeral. George was horrified that I intended to go but it's one of those things I feel I must do. An expression of solidarity. Feel sick, icy cold and only half there, but find the Church, know I'm in the right place when I see Sally and John who ask me to join them as I'm on my own. The service starts with the 23rd Psalm, Crimond, and after that I'm crying too much to register. So many people there from Clinic – Martha, Maxine, Drs Morrison and Keith, other parents. The flowers are lovely, a train, a teddy bear, a fire engine. Go with Sally and John to the cemetery where I can't stop shaking. Maxine comes and holds my arm. When I hug and kiss Betty and Frankie, he says How brave of you to come.

Sally and John take me back to the house with them. I'm in no state to drive myself anywhere. Dr Keith asks after Adam, says I'm not to worry about a simple cough (I'm not) but to bring him in straight away if he starts coughing blood, which could accelerate very quickly. That possibility just hadn't occurred to me. Drink coffee, itch to get back to Adam

– Sally asks John to drive me back to my car. Frankie hugs me, thanks me for coming, says they appreciate it a lot, can they have that dinner some time soon, and can they come to visit Adam.

Somehow I get home in one piece, go next door for Adam. Chris takes one look at me and fetches me a whisky. He says Adam's cough seems to have got worse during the afternoon but he isn't coughing anything up. Adam seems lethargic, mentions vague aches and pains he cannot specify but doesn't feel anything should be done about them. He doesn't know where I have been.

Concentrate hard on Positive Thinking, on relaxing; Adam and I tune in to one another, have a lovely evening together before I settle him happily into bed cuddling Roland Rat, with Cat at the foot of the bed.

Phone to cancel tomorrow's therapy appointment.

Tuesday 25 September

Adam starts the day quietly, livens up during the morning. We can't find the Snakes and Ladders counters among the deep-litter Lego on his bedroom floor, can't find a thimble even – so we play cards. Then Hunt-the-Dice, in lieu of a thimble. It's amazing how difficult it is to spot a dice even when it's red and quite obviously placed. We have a very good day together although I feel one step away from reality.

George didn't phone today either.

Wednesday 26 September

Adam doesn't wake or cough during the night but I'm somehow expecting him to, keep going through to look at him and spend a very restless night myself. After seeing to the animals, we play cards. How about that!

Thea comes to lunch, with a plant for me, sweets for Adam. She's so serene, smiling, familiar and understanding. Maxine arrives with two sorts of painkillers for Adam, some Gees Linctus for his cough which she says is better than the cough mixture I've been giving him. He tells her his right leg, the right side of his chest, the back of his neck hurt, but he doesn't want any tablets.

Thea amuses him while I talk to Maxine in the kitchen. She asks if I'd like a home help, having crunched across the floor;

decline with thanks, we don't want the fuss and bother. She says it's very unlikely that Adam would start coughing blood but it is possible. To phone Nick if he vomits or passes blood, or if I'm worried for any reason; to phone her day or night if there's anything I want to discuss. Remember they'll always have him on 4B if I need a break, even if he isn't having a crisis. She explains about the tablets – one or two Paramol every 4 hours for pain, and if that doesn't work use the stronger ones. She and Martha will come to lunch on Friday, she'll phone Nick and work out a support system with him so that one or the other of them visits every few days. God bless Maxine.

Thea too says she knows what I'm going through and to phone her day or night if I want to talk or if there is anything practical she can do. I have some beautiful friends.

Adam doesn't want lunch. When Thea leaves we play Hunt-the-Dice again which makes him laugh and laugh so much I can hardly believe he's ill.

Nick calls. Maxine hasn't reached him yet so I try to fill him in. He's so kind and supportive I can hardly believe it – he has hundreds of other patients too. He reiterates, call him any time, and he'll look in frequently too.

More games, see to the animals; amusing Adam again and thinking Positive Thoughts into him as we play – I'm exhausted by the time he's settled in bed.

George phones. I tell him Adam isn't too well and that the support he and I are getting from the medical people is superb. He doesn't seem to understand how much Maxine's and Nick's visits mean to me. Says he'll be here some time on Saturday.

Thursday 27 September

While Adam and I are playing cards this morning (is this addictive?) Louise's mother phones, another Clinic acquaintance – says she's heard from Sally about Adam's condition, has been thinking about us a lot and could she drop in for coffee. Lovely. She brings a posy of flowers from her garden, talks interestingly to Adam. I'm so warmed by people.

Just after she leaves Matron rings to tell me Grandad died peacefully in his sleep at 10:00 this morning, after being washed and tidied.

Tell Adam quietly. We agree we miss him – as he used to

be, not as he was during the last few months: as Adam says, he should have died before.

We sit quietly for a moment, contemplating, then Adam asks me what happens when you die. Don't know where it comes from, but I tell him it's a bit like baby chicks hatching – until they are ready to hatch they really need their eggshells and can't exist without them; once they are ready to come out they're free to live properly, enjoy their lives running around, and their eggshells are no use any more, like a body when the person inside has grown ready to leave it. He accepts this.

Adam wants to picnic so we pack up and drive around. We finish up at Brill once again, by the windmill, where we eat our picnic in the car, watch people walking dogs – in some cases it seems to be the other way around – and we walk a little, too, till Adam gets tired. Drive around some more, stopping when we see something we want to watch. Just little things. My mind is out of gear, I can't pray properly for Grandad. We come home, and play cards.

George phones from Heathrow to say his secretary reached him in Amsterdam with the news of his father, he'll be back shortly. What does one say, I can't tell him I'm sorry his father has died.

He sees a considerable change in Adam's appearance since last weekend.

Friday 28 September

George goes off to the nursing home and to see Mr Wilson the undertaker, while Adam and I play Ludo, Snakes and Ladders and – well, I'm tempted to hide the cards but he enjoys them so much.

Mix a salad for lunch. Maxine and Martha arrive, Adam shows Maxine his room while I tell Martha of my misgivings over poor Grandad's funeral. I should give George my support on such an occasion, people will come from quite a distance and I should offer them hospitality afterwards but I can't do it here. I've suggested George take a hotel room and get it all organised for us but he is as reluctant to do that as I am to leave Adam to attend the service.

Maxine comes down and says he's crying – apparently she asked if he'd been taking his tablets and he dissolved. Both she and I tell him no one is cross with him for not taking them, indeed if nothing hurts it's sensible not to take them, they are there so that he can have them if he does get a pain. How glad we are that there is no pain.

He won't come down to lunch with us but appears in a while to show them photographs and his plane book, talks to them while we all eat. Martha tells me several of the nurses on 4B who know Adam would be willing to come and sit with him, even stay the night, if I would like time off. What a comfort to know, but I can't imagine what I'd do with time off.

Maxine says she'd be happy to collect Adam, take him back to her house for a cup of tea to give me a chance to go to Grandad's cremation; she'll be in touch in a day or so. God bless Maxine.

They aren't here for very long but Adam becomes impatient for them to go so he and I can settle into playing again.

We are interrupted by a few phone calls about Grandad's cremation arrangements which is difficult because I don't want Adam to overhear anything – couldn't bear to have him around people getting over-emotional while he is so vulnerable.

My poor Adam looks terrible – white-faced with petechiae also on his face now, a fragile air about him, a clinging dependence on me. He enjoys our games very much though, and laughs a great deal. I Think Positive.

Saturday 29 September

Adam just wants lime juice for breakfast, nothing to eat. Play cards, watch television and cuddle till George arrives at lunch time. After lunch we go to Didcot, to the railway centre, wander around watching the beautifully-maintained old steam locomotives chuffing about. There's a lot to see, we all enjoy it, but Adam decides all too soon he's had enough, needs to go back. Put my arm around him, he stumbles a bit and we have to sit down to rest on the way back to the car. George is shattered.

Adam dozes on the sofa on our return, watching television. He grins persuasively at his father and asks for another Indian supper, eats very well and we have a good evening. How can we – what tenuous threads hold us together.

23

Sunday 30 September
Adam just eats potato for lunch, no meat or veg., maybe it isn't spicy enough for him. He bites around his thumbnail and it bleeds for four hours. He's cheerful and I work very hard at willing into him mental projections of love, security, serenity, while playing things like Ludo, I-Spy, whatever he wants.

Wherever did I get this mental projection stuff from?

George phones Victoria to tell her of her Grandad's death; she cries a lot although she has some idea of the state he was in. He plans to write to her saying Adam isn't too well but not to come home before planned.

He cuts the grass for me and goes back to London.

Monday 1 October
Adam spends the day in pyjamas and dressing-gown on the sofa and with his duvet over him, Cat next to him. Sit and love him, cuddle while we half-watch television. Which day was it he watched Let's Read with Basil Brush followed immediately by the birth of a baby, viewing both with equal interest?

When Maxine arrives late morning she stays with him while I rush to the bank and order flowers for Grandad's cremation. One lot from George and me; a posy from Vicki and Adam. God bless Maxine. She and I decide there is no point in taking him to Clinic tomorrow – it isn't worth the effort he would have to put into getting there. She'll phone Nick and tell him, she'll come again in a day or so, before then if I need her. She's such a comfort.

Adam is bothered because he's developed dandruff – Look, *snow* coming from my hair – nothing else worries him.

Sit next to Adam all afternoon, playing when he wants to, watching television, just cuddling him, trying to give him strength. Betty phones – they want to come over on Wednesday. I ask Adam, who says he'd like to see them. Explain to

Betty Adam isn't too good but they really want to see him.

He's gone down so much in the last few days it's unbelievable.

Tuesday 2 October

Check Adam so often in the night I end up in his room rather than mine. He's okay till early morning when I hear him retching in the bathroom and catapult out of my duvet – hold him while he tries to vomit but nothing comes up. He doesn't seem worried. Give him fresh cold water to drink.

It seems something about him has changed; ring Nicholas and ask him to look in on his way to the Health Centre. I couldn't say what has changed, but something has. Nick gives him a good going over and although his temperature is slightly up he can't find any localised reason to account for it, says it's just a general malaise because his white count is so low. We give him Stemetil to combat nausea, iced drinks to bring the temperature down. He positively refuses analgesics.

In fact he perks up quite soon, comes downstairs with his duvet and re-establishes residence on the sofa. With Cat.

Maxine phones to say she and Nick plan to arrive together around 12:30. Adam sleepy again. Nick prescribes morphine in small dose to stop anxiety feelings and more Stemetil syrup for nausea; Maxine fetches the prescriptions and also brings morphine ampoule and syringe, so everything is here if needed. Adam eats yoghurt, drinks a lot of lime juice.

The Vicar calls briefly and touches Adam's head; I'm sure he is silently blessing him again. Willow slips in with a big bowl of goose casserole with dumplings for me – no one else could possibly have neighbours like mine, the very word is heart-warming.

Primed by Willow, Phil calls during the evening to talk to Adam who, although he isn't exactly talkative, obviously enjoys seeing him. He thinks a lot of Phil. Karen walks in while Phil is here – both tell me I should get into the habit of shutting my door.

Persuade Adam to have one of his tablets – the doctor said it would make him feel better. He immediately throws it up again. He doesn't seem to be in pain or anxious. Help him have a bath, after which he pees, bright with blood. It doesn't hurt him, and I tell him it is just his body's way of getting rid of blood cells it doesn't need any more, quite calmly, and he accepts that. He doesn't need morphine, not him: I'm positive he is neither in pain nor anxious. When we've done teeth, said prayers together, kissed goodnight and settled him down, I go downstairs to Karen.

We have a drink, I tell her about the blood. She insists I phone Maxine, who says he'll probably pee blood all the time now, I can believe him when he says it doesn't hurt and am I okay? *Me?* Try to assure both Maxine and Karen that I don't fall apart at the sight of a little blood, but I do need to be reassured there's no pain.

Karen is almost out of petrol. It's a blessing that her car takes 2-star, of which I have a small store for the baby tractor. Around midnight we manage, by torchlight, to get most of a canful down the small funnel into her petrol tank and she goes home.

I've just gone upstairs when Adam tells me he peed blood again and he wants more lime juice. Tell him Maxine said that will probably happen now, and fetch him his lime juice. I spend the rest of the night on his bedroom floor. He is certainly not anxious about anything, he's far too relaxed. There's nothing at all in the air for me to pick up.

Wednesday 3 October

From 7:30 to 9:30 this morning poor Adam throws up two or three times – very little, but somehow we get through two duvet covers and three pairs of pyjamas; his bedroom carpet suffers too. He doesn't seem to feel bad and won't take any medicine, says he doesn't need it. He just wants iced water to drink so I can't slip anything into it. I ask if he'd like to go back to 4B; he says no, he wants to stay here with me and Cat.

Drape the sofa with soft towels and make him comfy with his sleeping bag over him; we watch television together. Maxine and Martha come over, Maxine bringing useful things like waterproof mattress cover, waterproof for the sofa, a bottle and a bedpan. However did she guess? I'm cuddling Adam, mopping his nose which is bleeding slightly.

Maxine sits with Adam while I hang out the washed duvet covers, sheets, etc. Martha comes out to join me, tells me I'm doing very well for Adam who is so calm and comfortable she can hardly believe it, and that it's a joy to see us together. I'm greedy for that sort of comment. Maxine says if Nick phones I'm to tell him there's been a change and maybe he'd like to look in. I saw a change yesterday morning – or rather felt one – but notice nothing different today.

Duncan arrives about 1:00 and comes through to see Adam, who says hello but not much else – he's happily watching television. Duncan follows me into the kitchen, hugs me and asks what the latest position is. He tells me the end will be very soon but that Adam is so peaceful and comfortable it's lovely, and I'm not to worry that he doesn't want his morphine. He decides that I should eat and wants to cook eggs for lunch – explain that I have some duck and orange soup ready from the freezer, all we have to do is turn it on and make some toast. He's most enthusiastic about the soup, says it's so good it must do Adam good, but Adam doesn't want any. I can't eat much, either, but Duncan does it justice. He holds my hands a moment, talks so kindly and hugs me again before he goes.

Willow comes in with a black toy cat to keep Adam company when Cat has to go out. He gives her a beautiful smile and cuddles it close.

It all sounds busy, but it isn't, it's very gentle, Adam-orientated, peaceful. A very special atmosphere. He doesn't want to play now, just lie, cuddling or holding hands, half-watching television, listening to Cat breathing.

Betty and Frankie arrive with a lovely natural history book for Adam, flowers for me. He doesn't say much but follows our conversation with interest, smiles a lot and murmurs yes or no occasionally. They are very kind, keep the conversation rolling easily in a quiet cheerful manner. I am painfully aware of how difficult this must be for them, but they insist they want to call again next week. Considerately, they don't stay long, either.

I go through to fetch Adam fresh iced water and find Dr Morrison coming in. He holds my hands and says quietly he doesn't think he'll see Adam again so he's called in to say goodbye. He comes through to the sitting room, strokes Adam's hands and his hair, speaks very kindly to him. He won't have a drink or anything, says he's on his way to give a lecture.

When Nick rings to ask how things are, would I like him to call in, I explain we've had visits from two consultant paediatricians today, and although things aren't good and Maxine said to tell him there had been a change, thank you but I don't think there is anything he could do. He'll call in the morning before surgery.

I can feel people's prayers and concern for us, giving us a strength so real it's almost visible. I'm sure we wouldn't be afloat without it.

George comes back early, 7:30, seems over-loud, larger than life for Adam and me; we've somehow geared down without realising it.

Adam seems so comfy on the sofa and he looks far too weak to manage the stairs, so he and I plan to stay downstairs tonight. After a couple of hours he shakes me by suddenly leaping up and saying, I'm going to bed now, striding briskly off up the stairs with me trotting after him, trying to catch up in case he becomes weak and falls.

Spend the night curled in my duvet on the floor of Adam's room again. He's restless, tossing and turning, wanting fresh iced water, wanting to pee. In between helping him, loving him, I lie there looking at him, trying to will in feelings of peace and security. I'm sure if I let go for an instant and my thoughts range wild, he'll pick up my fear of pain, fear of the unknown which faces us. I *have* to think good, positive things, to help both him and me.

The 23rd Psalm goes round and round in my head.

24

Thursday 4 October
This will be a dreadful day for poor George, going alone to his father's cremation. I don't want to add to his anxieties by telling him that I think we won't have very long with Adam now.

When Nick comes to see Adam he suggests we try to give him morphine in lime juice but he won't take it. I think we all want to give him morphine to alleviate *our* pain: he still says he has no pain. Thank God. He looks slightly jaundiced this morning, his face fuller, his eyes more bruised. Very sleepy, he decides to stay in bed.

The Vicar looks in for five minutes, blesses him again.

Willow has taken over the organisation of this afternoon, God bless her. She'll give them all tea, sherry and sandwiches in her house after the cremation service. I've apologised to George most sincerely and explained I can't leave Adam, even with Maxine, even to go with him to his father's cremation. I feel rotten about it, but there you are.

Pauline and Angela arrive early so they can say a quick hello to Adam, who isn't responsive. He tells me, no people, he just wants me and peace and quiet. We sit quietly together. He's still drinking a lot of iced water and his pee is less red now; he's pleased.

Sitting with Adam in his room, watching videos, trying to think good thoughts, yet feeling so badly for George that I can't be with him to pay my last respects to his father, I try to tell myself I did all I could for the old man while he was alive, having him here to live with me after mother-in-law died, then visiting and caring for him while he was in the nursing home. Do we ever feel we've done enough when someone dies?

George slips in from next door to ask if various people can come in to see us. Say no, thank them for their concern, but no. He meets Maxine during this interlude; she feels closer than most family, she's so dear to us, and she certainly doesn't count as a visitor. George goes back to talk to people and tell them Adam isn't strong enough for visitors.

Adam brightens up and asks where Daddy is – I say he had to go to a meeting and will be back soon. When he comes in, George insists on retuning the video and television, seems too large, too noisy in Adam's room. He goes back to London about 8:30.

Adam feels tickly, so I suggest sponging him down and changing him into fresh pyjamas; that idea is too undignified for him, he insists on getting up and having a bath.

He settles down and seems more peaceful than last night, although neither of us sleep much. My mind seems to have settled a little too. Suddenly as I'm lying there looking at him the most extraordinary thought comes into my mind: I'm ready now for you to leave me, my Adam. Amid trying to project concentrated dollops of love, peace and security, I send a mental message into his eyes, across all of three feet of floor space, saying, I know you have to go very soon, my Adam, you'll always be with me in a way, and you don't have to try to stay for me. I love you, Adam, I love you so much I can let you go. This is entirely involuntary and takes me by surprise, but I recognise the sentiments as genuine, really with love, peace and without fear. It's the most extraordinary feeling. I hope that I haven't held Adam with me for longer than was necessary for him, through the strength of my love for him perhaps getting slightly displaced. I pray for peace for Adam. For God's love for him. A strong, almost mystic feeling.

Friday 5 October
Adam drinks a great deal – I spend a lot of time fetching him fresh iced water. He watches a couple of videos in the morning, really participating, with laughter and his Pow! Pow! noises. Maxine and Martha come, sit quietly with him while I have a quick bath and change my clothes – I've been in the same clothes for three days and two nights. They are just leaving when Duncan arrives for some more duck and orange soup. He comes upstairs and sits with Adam and me for a little while, watching Star Trek. When the video needs changing Adam leaps out of bed to make sure I've put it in the right way up and pressed the right button – such energy!

He doesn't want us to eat in his room – the smell of food might make him feel sick, so Duncan and I have our soup in the dining-room. I'm constantly on the alert, checking Adam, but somehow manage to talk to Duncan, laugh with him even. His attitude makes me feel so much better, and he tells me I'm doing the right things, managing well for Adam . . .

Adam and I spend the afternoon quietly together watching television, apart from a quick visit from the Vicar, who again manages to put both his hands on Adam's head so I feel he's blessed once more.

This evening Chris and Willow look in to say they've just put the chicks and ducks to bed for me. Chris goes up to talk to Adam and they have a long and lively conversation while I thank Willow for all she did yesterday.

Nick rings to say he'll be away over the weekend, gives me two back-up names to call if need be. George comes at 9:30; Adam sleepy but very glad to see him. Give George scrambled eggs then he goes to bed. I once again curl up on Adam's floor in my duvet.

I'm in demand to provide fresh iced water, hold him and the bottle while he pees. We sleep for a couple of hours, Adam and I, then he starts to need things more frequently. Iced water, then to throw up a little, a bedpan. There's some blood in the vomit, a lot in the bowel movement; he doesn't notice and certainly doesn't seem distressed. By the time I have cleaned him and the receptacles, calmly and soothingly, he needs one of them again or more iced water. His nose is bleeding. Fetch an ice pack for the bridge of his nose. He's hot. For an hour I'm kept going at a steady pace doing things to help him feel comfortable, sponging his face, my mind saying, Darling Adam, you'll soon feel better, I'll make you feel better very soon. He insists he is not in pain, won't have analgesics.

At 3:00 a.m. he says he can't lie still, he's tickly, not comfortable. His breathing is shallow. He doesn't need anything for the moment, so I ask if he'd like me to ask Maxine if she knows of any way to make him feel more comfortable. He agrees, so I go through to wake George and ask him to phone Maxine. He says, At 3:00 – are you sure? Say, Yes, I'm sure it's all right, tell him what is happening and ask if he will report to her and see if she thinks it's time now to give the morphine injection. She apparently phoned Nick's substitute, who is here in ten minutes; Maxine herself is here from Oxford inside fifteen – do these people sleep in their clothes?

Both come in and sit on the floor in Adam's bedroom, watching him quietly. I'd wanted Maxine because not only do we know and love her, but she'd seen him earlier in the day, would in my opinion be more in a position to judge change than the doctor who has never seen him before; also she's experienced in this disease. Adam quietens a little. George is hovering outside the door, Adam suddenly says, Where's my Dad? I call and George is there instantly – lovely for them both.

The doctor and Maxine decide quietly to give Adam the diamorphine injection. Maxine slips it into his leg quickly while we hold each other tight; Adam relaxes almost instantaneously. His eyes don't quite close, he seems to be fighting sleep. I hold him, stroke him. George hauls Maxine out of the room to talk about Victoria; the doctor and I sit with Adam. Maxine returns, George went off to phone Justin's parents to tell them what is happening. I'm glad he has a phone call to make: he needs it.

The injection should be effective for about four hours, so when the doctor has made sure Adam isn't reacting badly to the first one, he makes arrangements for the weekend with Maxine, who says she'll stay with us now. He leaves, saying he'll look in after morning surgery and leaving a further ampoule with Maxine. Continue sitting by Adam, stroking him, with Maxine nearby.

Suddenly I decide to go change into my jeans – this is the first night for ages I've put on a nightie and it keeps tripping me up. Maxine taps on the bedroom door and calls through that Adam's breathing pattern has changed and his pulse is weaker. George and I jam in my bedroom doorway in our effort to get back to him. I hug Adam, hold one hand, pass the other to George. Stroke Adam's face, kiss him, tell him quietly and gently that I love him very much and he'll soon feel better, everything will be all right very soon my darling, I love you, over and over again. Adam's breathing gradually becomes less and less frequent. It isn't laboured in any way, he just doesn't want to do it as often. Maxine, curled up quietly on the floor at the foot of his bed, says gently, I think Adam is at peace now. It is 4:30 a.m., 6th October, 1984.

Saturday 6 October.
George makes coffee and brings up the whisky bottle too. We sit on the floor next to Adam; Maxine, George and I, drinking laced coffee. I smoke, too. How strange to be able to do these things, even to want to. We talk in whispers for some reason, as though he were asleep. Probably reassure one another that he wasn't in pain, I can't remember.

George goes off to phone Justin's father again, to tell him Adam has died. That makes it more real for him. I wash Adam – no, Adam's body – while George is out of the room. That makes it more real for me. Maxine helps. He's so heavy. We dress him in clean clothes, fasten his bunch of keys, his precious keys, to his belt. Maxine wants to phone the doctor to tell him Adam has died; I say, Why, there's nothing he can do now, there's no point in disturbing his sleep again, so we don't, although she thinks he would want to know. We have trouble keeping Adam's mouth closed and his eyes shut. She rolls up a pillow to push under his chin. It looks uncomfortable.

We go downstairs and drink more coffee. George and I try to thank Maxine for her kindness – such an inadequate word – and she says the experience has helped her a lot, this is the first time she has attended a child dying at home and how much nicer it is for the child. She thinks I managed well and that he wasn't in any pain or anxious at all – quite honestly I think he wasn't, too. She leaves around six in the morning.

George and I do mundane things between drinking more coffee. I put more washing into the machine, he lets out the chicks and ducks. He goes next door to tell Chris and Willow.

At 9:00 I walk down to the little shop to collect the newspaper and tell Olive that Adam died peacefully at home at 4:30 this morning. She's stunned, it wasn't a very nice thing to do to her. I hadn't thought of that, in my selfishness, just that through her the news would permeate the village. She cries, I don't, I hold her hands a moment, then walk back up the path feeling somehow conspicuous, rather like a character from High Noon waiting for someone to shoot me down. Phil stops to give me a lift, he's on his way to visit Adam he says. Tell him; he brings me home, has coffee with us; we try to thank him for the trips he took Adam on.

The doctor comes – Maxine phoned him at a respectable hour – looks at Adam's body and gives me the certificate to take to the Registrar of Deaths.

George is meeting the Vicar and Mr Wilson the undertaker this morning anyway, to inter his father's ashes in his mother's grave. Don't go along. Once again I feel very bad about it but can't leave my Adam alone in the house. Somehow it would feel even worse than leaving him with Maxine and going to the cremation. Feed Cat. Wish she could go with him. Give him the black toy cat Willow gave him instead, to comfort him. Put pennies on his eyes, two pennies each – they aren't heavy enough, these new ones. Sit with him until George brings the Vicar and Mr Wilson back.

I'm terribly civilised and give them sherry while they study their diaries and discuss funeral arrangements. The first date they suggest is George's birthday which isn't acceptable to me, so it's 12 October at 2:30. Home still seems to me to be the natural place for Adam to be, but not if it's going to upset people very much. They all feel strongly against it, say it's too long, so I agree Mr Wilson can come for him this afternoon.

Having rituals to follow is a great help. And constant repetition of the fact of Adam's death drums it into our minds firmly, wears down the resistance there.

George cries a little now and then. I don't: I feel almost euphoric that we managed this thing, Adam and I and our marvellous marvellous back-up team of medical friends and plain non-medical friends, as peacefully and comfortably for him as we possibly could; that there was no severe pain from pressure caused by bleeding in the joints or skull, no frightening haemorrhage, no interminable lingering in an increasingly distressed state. He was at home, with his father and friends around, his beloved Cat with him almost constantly, starting up her purr-motor when he stroked her; Adam and I, tuned in to each other, both able to laugh and enjoy things even during his last day. No hospital, drips, tubes, impersonal busy-ness, everything organised; at home.

George and I take it in turns to phone people. Find I am comforting them, telling them to talk to their husbands or wives, pour themselves a stiff drink, don't cry, it was all right.

Talking to Angela, who came up to my mother-in-law's funeral and to father-in-law's cremation just a few days ago, I find myself making the horribly sick joke that I should have asked the undertaker for family discount rates – how could I?

Maxine phones to ask how we are. However do you answer that?

Betty and Frank arrive unexpectedly. They've never met George. Strangely we all decide to go out to dinner, talk about our common experience – even though there are so many differences it's hardly a common experience. Somehow it turns into a highly-charged group therapy evening, an odd but very beneficial experience; wish I could explain it.

I sleep very well.

Later: Letters, phone calls, flowers arrive. Kind people offer help with funeral arrangements – someone will toll a bell, volunteers will give the Churchyard an extra tidy and cut the grass; village ladies will arrange extra flowers in the Church; Phil will direct parking.

George suffers strong guilt feelings, says he feels he let Adam down. Try to tell him guilt feelings are quite normal. When he asks me I have to admit I don't have any. Yet. My subconscience will undoubtedly dredge up something for me to feel guilty about; it's a very familiar state for me. Remind George of all the exciting things he gave Adam: holidays abroad, the boat trips, television games, plane flight; and that Adam had the more mundane things like picnics, zoo trips and card games from me anyway; he had the best of both worlds from two different people who both love him and whom he loved, instead of a double dose of the same sort of thing from similar personalities. I hope it comforts him. He keeps looking at me as though he expects me to explode at any moment. I still have a sense of achievement that we managed for Adam the greatest gift of life: an easy death.

We go along to the undertaker's, kiss Adam a last goodbye. I knew it of course but it's still a shock to feel his cheek refrigeration-cold. This isn't my Adam at all; my Adam has left. This is exactly what I am supposed to recognise just now, isn't it. I'm conforming.

George and I go shopping for something suitable for me to wear to Adam's funeral. Tell the woman in the shop I'm looking for something black or very dark grey, a dress or suit, size 12. No, I'm a size 10, she says. This is very nice, and fishes out an emerald green creation; or this, caramel, coral and green. Say no, those won't do, it's to wear to a funeral. Is it for evening? she says, flourishing something sequinned. *No, it's a daytime funeral.* How about this? She waves a wool dress mainly in that shade of yellow that makes my teeth hurt but mixed with red and – we're getting close – black zigzags on it. George and I can't look at each other by this time. I say with an awful clarity I want something to wear to my son's funeral. Do you have a black jacket, she says, this tartan skirt looks very nice with a black jacket. We can't get out of the shop fast enough.

Justin's parents are caring for Victoria beautifully. We've all agreed she'll stay in Australia for the time being: it'd be too much to ask her to fly home alone for her brother's funeral.

On one occasion during this week George asks if I'm all right. Say, No, I'm feeling a little wobbly. So he writes me out a cheque for £4,000. I appreciate the fact that he feels he wants to give me something; however it seems such a strange reaction to me, it feels rather like a child presenting you with his very precious dead frog. Wonder how he arrived at the amount. Feel incredibly cold and alone.

In the wine shop one day George is talking about five or six cases of this wine or that and I tell him sharply that we aren't having a party. Oh, he says, such and such a corporation want to send a representative, this company and that company. Tell him Adam is our child, not the Lord Mayor, and we don't need any representatives, just the people who knew him and were kind to him. At home again Willow comes in just as we are about to have a real fight over this; she and I sit and watch George composing the collage of photographs of Adam at all ages which I was going to make, while steam comes out of his ears.

George goes back to London at 8:30. I rush to phone my therapist who isn't there so I phone Ted and he comes round, bless him. Listens to me and somehow instils some courage and confidence so that I manage to stop feeling that I'll shoot George if he turns Adam's funeral into a party for his business associates and realise he of course feels the need of support from his friends too. God bless Ted and how could I have been so stupid?

The chief cleaner at the office phones to give me her sympathy and good wishes. She says they've all been so worried for us over the last year, but were told not to ring to ask me how things were going. I'm so glad she told me that: I'd been upset and hurt not to hear anything, having been connected with the firm in one way or another for many years. It also gives me a kick that it's the office cleaner who eventually has the nerve to defy instructions from on high, follow her instincts and ring me, while all those smart, decision-taking, business-suited individuals meekly do as they are told.

I have a burning need to say thank you to people for the trips and treats they gave Adam, the cards, letters and gifts they sent him, the support they gave George and me through visits, phone calls, prayers. Write some letters, also want to say something along those lines at the service; George says no, it'd make it emotional and upset people and *he* certainly couldn't do it. The funeral of a child *is* an emotional occasion; and I don't see why saying thank you for kindnesses should upset people, but perhaps it wouldn't be fair to George if I were to do that. The Vicar agrees to paraphrase what I want to say for me.

12 October

Don't know what to do with myself this morning.

I met George's friend Derek when he came to play the organ at mother-in-law's funeral. When he arrives to play for Adam's, looking absolutely grief-stricken, I go to meet him and say, We must stop meeting like this, which shocks him enough to break the ice. Go down and sit in the Church, absorb the atmosphere, while he and George play with the organ.

Pauline arrives early to give me moral support, makes me eat some paté and drink a glass of sherry. Dear Willow feeds George and Derek. I get dressed. Various other people arrive, ask if they can do anything. I don't even know what *I* should be doing. Liz and her ladies arrive, take over the kitchen, set out glasses and cups.

Go back upstairs, smoke and watch for the cars. When I see them I tell George – everyone else has gone on. He makes me wait a while before we set off in slow stately procession; he asks me to hold his hand. I watch the flowery car in front, tell myself it's Adam's eggshell, just his eggshell. Want to help guide the coffin into Church, George stops me. Try to concentrate on breathing deeply, steadily, without hyperventilating; stick my chin in the air.

The Church is full, a blur of faces I don't see. The Vicar is super, it seems a particularly moving service but maybe it always does. Flowers everywhere, so many flowers, so many people. Holding onto myself tight, so tight, saying politely, Thank you for coming, do come back to the house. Many do, and Liz and her ladies pass hot and cold food, drinks and tea. I try to say hello to everyone but I'm not registering, it's as though I'd been programmed, some sort of machinery set in motion which then just continues along the pattern. Don't feel anything.

People keep asking me what I'll do now. I don't know. Sleep. Tired, I'm so tired.

25

February 1986

Transcribing this has been an extraordinary experience. It comes almost as a shock to realise how early in the course of his illness and how clearly Adam told me he would die. If he knew during the later stages that he was indeed dying, he said nothing, although he had openings available when I told him of Dominic's death, and Grandad's. Maybe with his deep understanding of these things he considered it unnecessary.

And poor George, how very difficult and painful it all was for him. In a way it was easier for me because I could work actively at helping both Adam and Grandad; George remained in the spectator stands, without the contact with hospital staff, other patients; constant discussion and repetition of events and situations with such marvellous people as Duncan, Nick, Briony and Ted, which came my way and which helped me to become reconciled, insofar as I ever was, with the reality.

Why on earth didn't I record more detail of all the happy times – and there were so many intensely happy times – instead of simply saying so often we enjoyed this or that?

There are so many memories I want to polish up, but I don't want time to bend my memories, to turn Adam into something he wasn't. The difficulties and worries were an integral part of the child I love so much.

People keep asking me how I feel. Some, I think, really want to know. Mostly, they want to be reassured that I am 'over it', as though losing my son were nothing more than a bout of flu. I feel I am beginning to feel again, and it hurts.

Immediately after Adam's death I was partly emotionally-anaesthetised by shock (even though I was prepared for it) and partly euphoric that his life had ended without pain, without fear, peacefully at home. A deep and loving gratitude to the marvellous medical staff and friends who were so kind to him and who supported us both during the awful journey through his illness.

Then the euphoria went, leaving the emotional anaesthesia. An extensive void, a nothing-period. It seemed impossible that so many utterly unimportant things – the car, the washing-machine, a tree – could be tangible, functioning, viable things when Adam wasn't. Unreal.

George wanted to send me a long way away after Adam's funeral. The south of France, Florida, Australia – he thought I needed a complete change. I'm sure he was right, but there was nowhere I wanted to be, on my own. He needed to send me away so I compromised by going to a Health Farm for a few days. The treatments soothed away a lot of tensions – the massages were marvellous and the masseur said he was impressed with the mobility of my kneecaps; told him I'd spent a lot of time on my knees recently. I bet not many people manage to gain 4lb. on 1,000 calories a day for less than a week! It was a good idea, if somewhat unorthodox.

Told George that if he wanted to send me away it would seem more important to be somewhere other than home over Christmas; he arranged for Victoria to stay in Australia and for me to join her and my mother and brother there; he'd fly with me.

That was the first time I really cried for Adam – all the way from Heathrow to Singapore. Poor George.

I knew that visiting Australia would not be the holiday George thought it would be for me. The very fact of Christmas seemed insurmountable; meeting new people; telling my mother I didn't feel I could emigrate and live with her; it was a strain for a number of reasons but I climbed over Christmas, got through it all somehow.

When I returned home with Victoria in January I simply went into hibernation. Mental and physical exhaustion. I'd sit in bed for hours because I couldn't make up my mind which pair of dirty jeans to put on when I got up. There didn't seem to be anything to get up *for*, anyway. So cold, I thought I'd never feel warm again and it wasn't just the temperature, it was deep inside me. I only wanted to curl up small and nurse my pain. Only my tensions held me together. Plenty of things to do, no incentive to do them: opt out. Read a lot: escapism. Spend a lot of time in bed: seeking comfort and security.

Wearing Adam's shirts and sweaters, hearing his favourite songs on the radio, seeing his anorak hanging in the hall, his things around the house, even sleeping in his room, in the bed he died in, were comforting, reassuring things. The painful things I couldn't foresee, they jumped out at me unexpectedly. Fish fingers in the flotsam of the freezer; stopping for petrol and not having to buy crisps too; the house too tidy, too quiet; the things I no longer had to buy in the supermarket; waking in the night to find myself in his doorway and the shock of seeing his empty bed; the ache of not being able to touch him any more – we touched a lot, Adam and I; bouncing into the toyshop one day to buy a gift for a small visitor and suddenly finding it unbearable to be in there, rushing out shaking and in tears, without gift.

Victoria was super, so adult, so admirable I felt worse by comparison. She'd gone away a difficult teenager I had to work hard at understanding, and returned with the capacity to understand and make allowances for me while I took my turn at being difficult. She organised me, the shopping and cooking; I did as she told me. She was gentle, funny and sympathetically understanding, which made the very worst part absolutely terrible for me: I pray she never suspected how much I resented her for being alive when Adam wasn't. This feeling struck me hard, sharp and fast, was completely unexpected and so shameful I couldn't discuss it with anyone: I felt unnatural.

Life wasn't easy for her either. At home Adam's death assumed a reality for her which it hadn't had while she was in Australia. Partly to get her out of the house, I encouraged her to re-establish contact with old friends who invariably asked her, How's your little brother now? She would dissolve into tears and so would they. We discussed it, and decided the best thing to say was, Thank you for asking, Adam died in October, quite peacefully at home – he wasn't in any pain. She could cope with saying that, and if you thank people for wanting to know, tell them peace and no pain, they don't feel awkward about having enquired and the conversation can develop instead of grinding to a halt.

If you can get up and go to bed whenever you want to, do whatever you like, you go adrift on a sea of freedom and don't want to do anything. It's very constricting, too much freedom. I concentrated on trying to sublimate my spiky, resentful feelings and not a lot else for two or three months. Then, at the end of April, I stopped being able to visualise Adam only after death, began to see him happy and laughing again. That was a tremendous release and somehow allowed me to appreciate my poor Victoria again, to enjoy her for herself.

She started a job in London, living with her father during the week, coming home to me at weekends. We could talk about Adam or not, quite naturally. She helped me go through his things; some we gave away, some we kept.

One day I bought a piece of furniture and some curtain fabric – felt very pleased with myself for making positive decisions on my own initiative. It made me feel a person in my own right, not just a redundant wife and redundant mother. Such a little thing but it felt like a big step forward.

I felt ready to branch out, decided that, although it might be nice to spend the summer drifting, getting the garden into shape, it would help me through the next winter if I were to organise myself now. Adam once asked me what Mrs X was *for* – she didn't go out to work or have children to look after, so what was she there *for*? I had sufficient ego to believe I was *for* something: it was time I tried to find out what.

I'd always had someone to take care of. Think about it deeply, but decide I couldn't bear to foster a child, I'm just not big enough.

Needed commitments to give my life a structure, needed to feel useful, needed people. Start dabbling my toes in a few local projects to see if anything will spring out as of overwhelming interest, whether I can make myself useful. Enjoy doing those things, meeting new people, inviting old friends over; felt everything was going well, I was under control, coping sensibly.

Now, I'm relapsing. I do not understand why, when it comes to the point of doing something, I'm quite likely to disintegrate into a small heap of insecurity, drenched in cold perspiration, shaky, cold clammy hands and feet, feeling I'm only safe at home and I want everything to stop. I'll feel convinced no one really wants my company or opinions, they just put up with me because they're sorry for me; I'll feel sure I'll forget how to do something basic like driving or having dinner ready when I've invited people over. I do these things without mishap but it all becomes such an effort it's exhausting rather than a pleasure.

I know perfectly well it's natural to feel extremely low sometimes because I miss him so dreadfully. I still wake up in Adam's doorway some nights, still come into the house wanting to tell him about the little things which would make him smile, like the beautiful sinuous grass-snake with her bright yellow collar which I almost picked up by mistake near the duckpond; the thrush so determined to finish tugging his worm out of the lawn that I had to stop the baby tractor and wait for him.

I miss both my children. Victoria is simply no longer a child. While obviously I'm still deeply concerned for her well-being, our relationship has changed and I recognise her as an independent individual who needs to leave home, and the easier I make it for her to go, the more free she will feel to come back to me. I don't want to smother her by over-protectiveness or over-dependence. Indeed I have to adjust to a whole new way of life. Not so long ago I had a husband, two children, a father-in-law and a variety of dependent animals to care for; now there's only Cat and me.

I think I'm doing the right things, so why these frightening panic, lack of self-confidence attacks? It's so stupid. Is it because I *can* now feel capable, independent and happy sometimes that the low periods hit me so hard I feel something must snap? Am I trying too hard, pushing too much, too soon? Maybe I have to go through these doubts, guilts and lack of confidence feelings in order to allow my emotions time to catch up at last with what I know, quite clearly, intellectually. But I don't understand the time-lag. Martha and Maxine think I came a long way in a very short time and a bit of back-sliding, although tough, is natural.

I feel I should have learnt something from all this, should be able to put it to some use to justify it. It's still bewildering. Many people have told me I must not expect to feel anything like normal for at least two years. Maybe some time, somewhere, it will all make sense.

ELIZABETH WARD

TIMBO: A STRUGGLE FOR SURVIVAL

Many people in Britain today carry a kidney donor card, yet few probably have any idea how, where or why the practice originated. TIMBO, A STRUGGLE FOR SURVIVAL is the personal story that lies behind these cards.

In September 1966, Elizabeth Ward suddenly discovered that her 13-year-old son Timbo had developed a severe kidney problem. It was a discovery that changed the lives not only of the Ward family but of thousands of kidney sufferers throughout Britain, and led to the founding of the British Kidney Patient Association in 1975.

But for Elizabeth Ward, the constant deterioration of Timbo's health was the most painful way to learn about any disease. Together they fought against hospitals, failed transplants, a lack of public awareness, and the disease itself. This book is the story of that struggle.

'Fascinating reading on both human and ethical grounds'
Good Housekeeping

'A story that tugs the heart'
Church Times

'A harrowing and heroic story ... an inspiring example'
Emlyn Williams

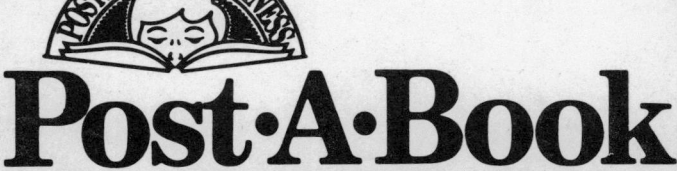

Post·A·Book

A Royal Mail service in association with the Book Marketing Council & The Booksellers Association.
Post-A-Book is a Post Office trademark.

MORE TITLES AVAILABLE FROM HODDER AND STOUGHTON PAPERBACKS

☐ 42595 9	**ELIZABETH WARD** Timbo: A Struggle for Survival	£2.95
☐ 41008 2	**TERESA McLEAN** Metal Jam	£2.95
☐ 40861 8	**POLLY TOYNBEE** Lost Children	£3.50

All these books are available at your local bookshop or newsagent, or can be ordered direct from the publisher. Just tick the titles you want and fill in the form below.

Prices and availability subject to change without notice.

Hodder & Stoughton Paperbacks, P.O. Box 11, Falmouth, Cornwall.

Please send cheque or postal order, and allow the following for postage and packing:

U.K. – 55p for one book, plus 22p for the second book, and 14p for each additional book ordered up to a £1.75 maximum.

B.F.P.O. and EIRE – 55p for the first book, plus 22p for the second book, and 14p per copy for the next 7 books, 8p per book thereafter.

OTHER OVERSEAS CUSTOMERS – £1.00 for the first book, plus 25p per copy for each additional book.

Name ....

Address ....

....